RB 36.3 .P55 M43 1985

Medical laboratory planning
and design

DATE DUE

DEMCO 38-297

MEDICAL LABORATORY PLANNING AND DESIGN

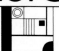

MEDICAL LABORATORY PLANNING AND DESIGN

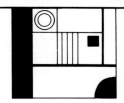

Compiled by the
LABORATORY FUNCTION AND DESIGN COMMITTEE

A. SAMUEL KOENIG, M.D., *Chairman*

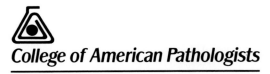

College of American Pathologists

Second Printing, 1989

Third Printing, 1992

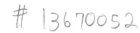

Library of Congress Catalog Card Number: 84-072829
ISBN: 0-930304-25-X
Printed in U.S.A.

*"Experience is not what happens
to you; it is what you do with
what happens to you."*

—ALDOUS HUXLEY

PREFACE

The concept for this book originated several years ago from James D. Barger, MD, who was then president of the College of American Pathologists. Jim noted that many medical laboratories in the United States were reminiscent of college chemistry student laboratories in layout, construction, and esthetics. He wondered if a book could be produced which would address the design problems of the modern medical laboratory and at the same time emphasize that laboratories should be functional and esthetically pleasing. Jim's desire has been confirmed by the many calls the CAP receives each year from individuals requesting assistance in medical laboratory planning and design. To this end, I was asked to undertake the task.

Having experience in the laboratory planning and design process personally, it seemed clear that one of the biggest problems hurdled by any pathologist engaged in planning and design, is an understanding of the process itself. So frequently there is a lack of informed communication and understanding between the pathologist, architect, and administrator. It seemed futile to produce a book written by pathologists and for pathologists when they must communicate their design needs to others inexperienced in the problems and concepts of medical laboratories. Most pathologists also lack knowledge of the architectural process. Therefore, it seemed much more reasonable to undertake the task as a collaborative effort of pathologists, chemists, architects, planners, and administrators.

Contact was made with the American Institute of Architects (AIA) and they were invited to participate in this project by appointing a task force composed of architects, engineers, and planners experienced in the design of medical laboratories. The AIA was most receptive to this invitation and several of their members were subsequently appointed to the group by the AIA Committee on Architecture for Health. Additional individuals, representing the American Association of Clinical Chemistry and hospital administration, were invited to join in the task. With the formation of the group thus completed, we began in

May 1982. As might be expected, we required some period of time to get on the same "wavelength," but it was clear to me early that this was truly a "blue-ribbon" group.

It became the fervent desire of the group to produce a book addressed to both pathologists and architects. We wanted it to serve as a bridge of knowledge and understanding between these two groups. In addition, we wished to avoid the material becoming rapidly dated. To this end, we tried to emphasize the *process* of planning and design. We also wanted to point out the unique knowledge base each party brings to the basic planning and design process. The organization of this book is an attempt to emphasize this fact, i.e., at which point in the planning and design process each area of expertise is used.

This proved to be an enjoyable learning experience for all of us. It is our sincere desire that you, the reader, will find our efforts useful and long lasting.

A. S. KOENIG, MD

CAP LABORATORY FUNCTION AND DESIGN COMMITTEE

A. SAMUEL KOENIG, MD, *Chairman*
LARRY D. SHAW, MD, *Vice-chairman*
S. STEVEN BARRON, MD
ALFRED E. HARTMANN, MD
GLENN M. MARTIN, MD
EDWARD W. BERMES, PhD, *AACC Liaison*
ARTHUR G. GARIKES, *Consultant*
ROBERT HABIG, PhD, *AACC Liaison*

AIA COMMITTEE ON ARCHITECTURE FOR HEALTH TASK FORCE

K. SHAHID RAB, AIA, *Co-chairman*
LEONARD MAYER, *Co-chairman*
JOHN J. CUMMISKEY
EDWIN LEVENTHAL, PhD

CAP STAFF

PAMELA CRAMER
ALISON WALLACE
NANCY KASNER

CONTRIBUTORS

S. STEVEN BARRON, MD
Grant Hospital
Chicago, IL 60614

JOHN J. CUMMISKEY, AIA
MEDIFAC
Pennsauken, NJ 08110

ARTHUR G. GARIKES, AIA
Garikes and Partners, Architects, Inc.
Health Facilities Planning Associates, Inc.
Birmingham, AL 35203

ROBERT L. HABIG, PhD
Duke University Medical Center
Durham, NC 27710

ALFRED E. HARTMANN, MD
Physician's Laboratory
Sioux Falls, SD 57105

MICHAEL D. HELM
Sparks Regional Medical Center
Fort Smith, AR 72901

A. SAMUEL KOENIG III, MD
Family Medical Care
Fort Smith, AR 72901

ALASTAIR G. LAW
MMP International Inc.
Washington, DC 20007

EDWIN A. LEVENTHAL, PhD
Friesen International
McLean, VA 22101

GLENN M. MARTIN, MD
Royal Inland Hospital
Kamloops, BC
Canada V2C 2T1

LEONARD MAYER, AIA
Lark IV Associates, Ltd.
Alexandria, VA 22314

K. SHAHID RAB, AIA
Northeastern Architecture
VA Medical Center
Washington, DC 20420

LARRY D. SHAW, MD
Senora Laboratory Sciences, Inc.
Mesa, AZ 85202

TABLE OF CONTENTS

INTRODUCTION

This book is written for all of those interested in medical laboratory planning and design, but most especially the pathologist and architect. The organization is somewhat unique, and to benefit fully, the reader should pay particular attention to the following comments on the organization of the book.

The organization emphasizes the *process* of medical laboratory planning and design and the knowledge base that is brought into each step of the process. To illustrate this further there is a common diagram that appears at the beginning of each part. This diagram shows the reader where each chapter fits into the whole process and knowledge base of laboratory planning and design.

The book is divided into five major parts. Each major part is presented in the sequential steps of the planning and design process. The first chapter of each part represents the major discussion of that step of the planning and design process. For an understanding of the basic overall process of planning and design, the reader should read in sequence the first chapter of each part of the book. The subsequent chapters in each part represent various areas of knowledge base that come into play or impact on that step of the planning and design process. These "knowledge base" chapters are further separated on the diagram into laboratory and architect/planner areas of expertise. Each of the chapters stands alone and may be read as such.

Both pathologists and architects will find useful the section pertaining to preparation for the planning and design process. It represents basic background information and philosophy of approach that everyone should be familiar with.

The laboratory knowledge base chapters are of greatest use to architects. Pathologists will find them elementary, but should skim the material at least. The converse is true of the architect/planner knowledge base chapters.

The reader is encouraged to approach the book in the manner he finds most comfortable—but is encouraged to read it all!

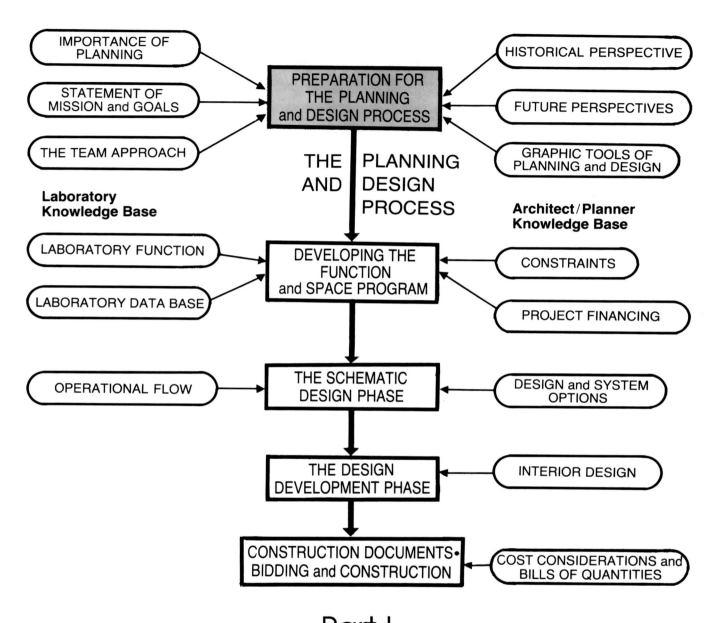

IMPORTANCE OF PLANNING

STATEMENT OF MISSION and GOALS

THE TEAM APPROACH

HISTORICAL PERSPECTIVE

FUTURE PERSPECTIVES

GRAPHIC TOOLS OF PLANNING and DESIGN

PREPARATION FOR THE PLANNING and DESIGN PROCESS

THE PLANNING
AND DESIGN
PROCESS

Laboratory Knowledge Base

Architect / Planner Knowledge Base

LABORATORY FUNCTION

LABORATORY DATA BASE

DEVELOPING THE FUNCTION and SPACE PROGRAM

CONSTRAINTS

PROJECT FINANCING

OPERATIONAL FLOW

THE SCHEMATIC DESIGN PHASE

DESIGN and SYSTEM OPTIONS

THE DESIGN DEVELOPMENT PHASE

INTERIOR DESIGN

CONSTRUCTION DOCUMENTS• BIDDING and CONSTRUCTION

COST CONSIDERATIONS and BILLS OF QUANTITIES

Part I

PREPARATION FOR THE PLANNING AND DESIGN PROCESS

cies in determining regulations are the present and projected increased costs of health care. Diagnosis Related Groups (DRGs) and Prospective Payment Systems are being implemented under new Medicare regulations. Other proposals, such as competitive bidding, uniform fee schedules, Health Maintenance Organizations (HMOs), and Preferred Provider Organizations (PPOs) may alter significantly the money available for laboratory operation and construction. The effect of these changes in health care payment cannot be predicted with certainty at this time, but the net result may be fewer tests performed, fewer test profiles, more organ panels and discrete tests, and new interpretive reporting systems. Preadmission testing will be more common. All but emergency laboratory testing may be performed outside of the hospital by large commercial and regional laboratories. The result is that hospital laboratories may become smaller, ceasing to show the steady growth in size, equipment, and test volume that has existed previously.

Considering these uncertainties, maximum flexibility of design and function is mandatory. These and other factors highlight the necessity for the construction or remodeling plan to incorporate the lowest reasonable cost for initial design and construction. The resulting laboratory must be capable of functioning economically when in operation. In the future, medical laboratory design must incorporate the potential for flexibility to respond to change at low cost.

This potential for flexibility can be enhanced by open laboratory plans, rather than small isolated units with fixed walls. Flexible modular furniture and casework can be relocated and reorganized easily and economically to meet future changes. Functional relationships must be considered both within each laboratory section and the laboratory's relationship to its service milieu. Most importantly, the design should be sensitive to the human needs of physicians, laboratory staff, and patients. This sensitivity includes a pleasant, attractive, esthetic environment, adequate work space, safety, suitable lighting, ventilation, air-conditioning, and humidity and noise control.

Functional and physical relationships to other hospital sections such as the operating, delivery, and emergency rooms, outpatient section, and intensive care units should be considered in the planning process. The plans should include specimen flow, planning for new admission testing, blood donors, outpatients, and turnaround time requirements. Several examples are given here, and more detail follows in other chapters. The various units of the laboratory should be located to minimize traffic congestion. Specimen receiving and sorting

" . . . The design needs of each laboratory are unique for the personnel and services it must provide. "

areas should be positioned near the specimen flow entrance to the laboratory, with logical progression to the various laboratory sections and work units for processing. The plan should restrict entry into the laboratory by nonlaboratory personnel. Phlebotomy units for outpatients should be in the outpatient area. For ambulatory inpatients, the phlebotomy site should be near the entrance to the laboratory area. If possible, night activity areas in each laboratory section should be concentrated near each other, to avoid unnecessary long distances to be covered by the night shift personnel. With an open floor plan, this concentration of equipment for maximum efficiency is more feasible for both daytime and nighttime uses. Within each area and laboratory unit, concentration of space, equipment, and personnel enhances efficiency.

The design needs of each laboratory are unique for the personnel and services it must provide.

DEVELOPING A STATEMENT OF MISSION AND GOALS 2

THE STEADY GROWTH of hospital and particularly laboratory facilities in the decades following World War II was often a situation in which planners, architects, and pathologists rushed to compensate the obvious inability of space in laboratories to meet workload demands. Planning, as we now understand the term, was either nonexistent, shortsighted, or based on simple rules of thumb. No matter how well intentioned, previous planning of laboratories now is recognized as being inadequate for the purpose of positioning the laboratory properly for its future. True, the prediction of the future is at best a process fraught with difficulties and uncertainties. Nonetheless, the current theory of planning, sometimes called strategic planning, requires an organized and thorough investigation of the following questions before embarking on a building program:

- *Where are we and how did we get here? (This is the situation analysis.)*
- *What is the external environment of the future (a specific period e.g., ten years) going to be like?*
- *What do we choose for our mission and goals in this future?*

The specific laboratory project that develops from such a planning process is presumed to have a better chance of being appropriate than the previous demand-pushed expansions.

The situation analysis for a laboratory should include an identification of the functions the laboratory performs, and a judgment of whether these functions are being performed the way they should be. It is reasonable to stop considering these functions after one has identified those that account for 80 percent to 90 percent of the workload, which may reduce the overall list of hundreds of functions to 20 or 30 functions. The situation analysis also should identify the competitors, those organizations that actually or potentially perform the same

5

services as the laboratory, and evaluate the strengths and weaknesses of these competitors. Like the practice of primary medicine, which has evolved from a single form, private practitioner and patient, to a multiplicity of forms, i.e., group practice, HMO, and PPO, laboratory medicine is now practiced in a variety of forms, each of which has to be considered and evaluated before beginning a major bricks-and-mortar project.

This complicated analysis is not all that needs to be done. The future, which once seemed to follow simple straight-line projections, is now cloudier than ever. Demographic patterns shift rapidly; government regulations shift incentives; and technological advances proceed at an accelerating rate. An investigation of the opportunities and threats (as projected into the defined future) is required. The prudent planner makes an effort to construct a scenario for the future and fashions his role and his actions to be consistent with that scenario and to protect against alternate outcomes whenever possible. In projecting the future, help is available from professional organizations, colleagues, writers, and commentators.

Finally, the organization or practitioner is ready to select the role and mission in the unfolding sequence of the future. The laboratory may continue the same way as it has been or it may become more or less automated, more or less centralized, or more or less specialized. It may tighten or loosen affiliation with institutions. *Choices made at this point set the course for the entire planning and design process that this book addresses.* To paraphrase a thought that Lewis Carroll expressed many years ago, if you don't know where you want to go, then it doesn't much matter which road you take. The task is not overwhelming. If the necessary aptitude for listing and organizing is not at hand, professional planners are available.

An example of a **mission statement** for a hospital-affiliated clinical laboratory might be

> "The mission of this laboratory is to perform analytical tests and provide diagnostic and therapeutic laboratory services on behalf of both inpatients and outpatients at Community Hospital and residents of Center City, Kansas, and the doctors that treat them. These services shall include all the regular laboratory services normally provided to patients, except that we will not offer services for autopsies, whole blood collection, or virology. Services are to be performed to the highest available standards for accuracy and are to be provided in a timely fashion in order not to delay diagnosis and treatment."

A **goal** for this laboratory might be

> "To attract new patients and doctors such that five years from now,
> 60 percent of the clinical laboratory services required in Center City
> are performed in our laboratory."

A **second goal** might be

> "To automate 70 percent of the workload."

Note that the mission statement may contain some generalities or idealistic qualifiers; the goals should be precise and realistically attainable.

Clearly, even specific goals will not contain sufficiently detailed information to guide the balance of the planning and design process. However, these goals set the major framework for the goals of the individual laboratory subunits, and establish a measure for the subunits' goals. The design process is then guided by the larger set of goals that includes all the laboratory units.

This is the latest concept of long-range, or strategic planning, as it is being used by private companies and major instutions worldwide. Each laboratory director should be aware of this methodology and apply it to the director's process of planning. Ultimately, the mission and goals become a unique statement reflecting the desires and judgments of their creators.

THE TEAM APPROACH TO DESIGN 3

THE CREATION OF A NEW LABORATORY or the renovation of an existing laboratory begins as a planning project and evolves into an architectural project. The architectural project is further divided into two phases: design and construction. The planning and design of a laboratory requires the involvement of four major parties:

- *Planner*
- *User*
- *Architect*
- *Owner*

In the case of a hospital laboratory or large regional laboratory, the owner most often is the community, government, religious order, or professional corporation. For most activities the owner is represented by the administrator/director. For a major design and construction project, a Board of Trustees or its equivalent group may appoint a building committee to work with the architect and oversee the construction project.

Pathologists and laboratory personnel are the users. The pathologist should represent the user. In the case of a private laboratory owned by a pathologist, the owner and the user are the same. However, in a larger sense the user is a broad spectrum of people including the clients who send specimens to the laboratory and patients.

The architect is hired by the owner for the design of a new laboratory or for renovation of an existing laboratory. The architect represents a design team incorporating a number of disciplines: architecture, planning, landscape architecture, interior design, and mechanical/electrical/civil/structural engineering.

> " *. . . The laboratory planner may be an inhouse planning group, consultant, pathologist, or an architect . . .* "

9

A laboratory planner may provide valuable support to the team. The laboratory planner may be an inhouse planning group, consultant, pathologist, or an architect commissioned to perform planning studies. The planning architect may be the same architect commissioned to provide the design services.

Roles of the Major Team Members

The Laboratory Planner

The planner can perform or assist the owner and user in the following services:

- *Programming*
- *Equipment selection*
- *Follow-up and coordination*
- *Staffing patterns*
- *Project and construction costs*
- *Dealing with regulatory requirements*

Writing a program (see glossary), which includes determination of functional and space requirements for the laboratory, is the most important task before the design of the laboratory can begin. The planner may determine expected patient/service requirements for the target year, which could extend five years or more into the future. Demographic studies, service area, or market analysis data may be needed in order to project future changes in the patient/service volume. Often these items of information can be found in a well-documented, long-range plan for the institution. Based on the projected service requirements and the method of working in the particular laboratory, the planner can derive a reasonable laboratory space requirement. This is one of the most difficult tasks of laboratory planning.

No universally accepted method of determining space requirement exists. In 1981, Health and Welfare Canada took a bold, but limited, step in coming up with a preliminary relationship between workload and space requirement. The suggested range for the total laboratory is 4,950 to 6,670 workload units per gross square meter. This is the average for the total laboratory; there are different values for the various sections within the laboratory. In many countries of Europe and Asia where health care is partially or totally socialized, space standards for different levels of laboratories exist, i.e., community, district, and regional. However, these are not applicable to North American laboratories. The experienced planner knows that the space requirement of the laboratory is a function of not just the workload, but of factors such as working methodology in the particular laboratory, staff size, and additional services of teaching, consultation, infection control, and community programs.

The planner should discuss possible changes in working methodology with the pathologist in order to improve space efficiency. One example of such change is to increase automation.

The experienced laboratory planner can assist the pathologist and the architect in the selection of equipment. Laboratory equipment can be divided into two categories:

" . . . No universally accepted method of determining space requirement exists."

1. Instruments and laboratory equipment that are used to perform the test procedures. These items consist of such things as analyzers, refrigerators, centrifuges, etc. The pathologist will have primary responsibility in the selection of such instruments and equipment.

2. Fixtures and furniture that create the working environment. These include casework, tables, chairs, cold rooms, moveable partitions, etc. The architect has the responsibility to assist the user in the selection of this equipment.

The planner can provide equipment recommendations to both the user and the architect, coordinate space and equipment, and provide the architect with the environmental requirements of the equipment.

During the design phase, the planner can provide on-going review of architectural drawings to ensure that the programmatic space requirements and functional relationships are met. If the planner is also a specialist in laboratory planning and design, the planner can provide valuable assistance to the architect and user by providing detailed and in-depth information on laboratory systems, operation, and equipment.

During the design process it is the architect who bears the statutory responsibility and liability for the design of the laboratory. Therefore, the architect reserves the right to be selective about implementing the planner's recommendations.

The planner can provide follow-up and coordination. The total time span between the beginning of planning and the completion of construction may be several years. If the laboratory being constructed is part of a major medical center, the time span may be as long as ten years. Therefore, laboratory communication systems and equipment needs should be reviewed and updated at appropriate intervals. Update and change involving elements of the building should be completed during the architectural design development phase. Other equipment changes can take place as late as the construction phase, ensuring that the newest developments in equipment are considered. The planner can provide on-going monitoring service and initiate the updating process by bringing significant information to the attention of the pathologist and architect. Post-construction and post-occupancy reviews for the facility are additional services that may be provided by the planner.

If requested by the owner, the planner works with the owner and user to develop staffing patterns for the new laboratory facility. In doing this, the experienced planner points out the pros and cons of the following and other factors affecting staffing:

- *Workload and service requirements*
- *Hours of operation*
- *Automation*
- *Functional layout of the laboratory*
- *Specimen transport system*
- *Information processing system*
- *Ratio of full-time, part-time, and on-call technical personnel*
- *Teaching and research responsibility of the laboratory*

One key service that may be provided to the owner by the planner is an idea of the project cost at an early stage of the project. The owner may have to adjust the scope of the project based on this information. The planner can explain the difference between project and construction costs. Project cost includes construction costs plus costs of land, fees, equipment, financing, salaries of owner's personnel involved in the project, etc. Cost figures provided by the planner are preliminary and provide the owner with a rough idea of the cost of the project. More accurate estimates are provided by a professional cost estimator or quantity surveyor through the architect. The final construction cost figure is provided by the contractor at the time of bidding.

The planner may assist the owner in dealing with regulatory and health planning requirements. An important step may be to obtain a Certificate of Need. Requirement of regulatory agencies for design and construction related items, such as meeting fire and safety codes, and obtaining building permits, generally will be handled by the architect and contractor.

The User

For purposes of planning and design the laboratory staff represents the user. This group of people includes pathologists, other MDs, PhDs, technologists, phlebotomists, clerks, and secretaries. The user generally provides the following services to the design team:

- *Need determination and project initiation*
- *Laboratory long-range or master plan*
- *Laboratory work flow and data base*
- *Liaison with other sections*
- *Selection of design options*
- *Project manager*
- *Consultant selection*

The pathologist, as the laboratory director, has a key role in need determination and initiating the planning and design project. It is true that the owner, for example, represented by the hospital administrator, may sense the need for expansion/renovation of the laboratory. It is the pathologist, however, being the day-to-day occupant of the facility, who knows all the shortcomings of the existing facility and who can articulate the need for a new facility or for expansion and/or renovation. When the planner is engaged to determine the need more precisely, the pathologist can assist the planner by providing workload data and by explaining the mission and working methodology of the laboratory. Based on his daily experience in the laboratory, the pathologist is able to explain the qualitative and quantitative effects of constraints on space and equipment. The owner, planner, and architect all need to be aware of these. A good understanding of the problems by everyone leads to good solutions.

The pathologist should participate in the preparation of the long-range or master plan of the laboratory. More often than not, a master plan is prepared for the larger institution, such as a hospital, of which the laboratory is a part. However, it always helps if the laboratory has its own long-range plan, which can then be placed into the master plan of the total institution.

The pathologist knows the work flow and data base of the laboratory.

" . . . The pathologist, as the laboratory director, has a key role in need determination and initiating the planning and design project."

13

These and the desired or expected changes in them should be explained to the other team members. The planner and architect bring ideas based on their experience in other laboratory projects. The pathologist should be willing to listen to these ideas.

Except in the case of a free-standing laboratory, planning, design, and operation will have significant impact on other sections and how medicine is practiced in the larger setting. Similarly, other sections will impact on the laboratory. Many times during the project, combined meetings of representatives from a number of sections will be needed to resolve such issues as:

- *Specimen collection*
- *Specimen transport*
- *Turnaround time for tests*
- *STAT laboratory capabilities*
- *Relationships between the laboratory and other hospital departments*

The pathologist has a major role in evaluating design options presented by the architect. In the case of a hospital laboratory, the hospital administration should rely almost totally on the judgment of the pathologist in the selection of design and operational options, as long as the laboratory remains within the programmed space and its design is not in conflict with the design principles of the total institution. Many facility systems the laboratory will use are hospital-wide. These may include a large-item transport system, a small-item transport system, computer system, and telephone and intercom system. The needs of the laboratory should be explained in detail to the architect so the requirements of the laboratory can be integrated into the overall plan. Insistence on a unique system just for the laboratory is probably going to be a mistake.

The pathologist should function as the official laboratory project manager and coordinate and collect the staff input for transmission to the architect. In a large laboratory the task of coordination may be delegated to a technical supervisor of the laboratory who may act as a moderator in work sessions between the representatives of various sections of the laboratory and the architect.

The pathologist should be involved in the selection of consultants. The consultant may be either a generalist or a specialist. In a hospital project that includes the laboratory as one of the components, a generalist, i.e., a hospital consulting firm, would be a good choice. Such a firm would have personnel with various levels of experience in dealing with the many functions in the hospital.

The Project Architect

The architect is responsible for the following project phases which are detailed in later chapters.

- *Schematic design*
- *Design development*
- *Construction documents*
- *Bidding or negotiation*
- *Administration of the construction contract*

The architect also offers occupancy and post-occupancy review as additional services.

The Owner

The owner of the facility is the official client and brings the following services to the planning and design team:

- *Project development*
- *Space allocation*
- *Long-range planning*
- *Financing*
- *Project oversight*
- *Liaison with board, community, and agencies*
- *Consultant selection*
- *Conflict resolution*

Laboratory project development may be initiated by a hospital administrator or by a pathologist owner. The owner engages an architect or planner, or both, to start the planning and design process. Depending on the protocol of the institution and the size of the project, the administrator may need authorization from a Board of Directors before engaging the architect. Once the project begins, the owner is involved in making decisions at every phase of the project.

A key role for the owner is to act as a referee for space allocation. In a hospital setting the pathologist is concerned with the space for the laboratory, while the administrator is concerned with the space needs for the whole hospital. If the project involves a number of sections, and the construction budget is tight, even the most thoroughly documented requirements for the laboratory may need to be cutback.

Along with the immediate project at hand, the owner focuses on the long-range plan for the whole facility. The owner also assesses how the present project fits into and impacts the long-range plan. Every single project may not fit perfectly within the long-range plan. Some projects may have to be done for temporary expediency, only to be drastically modified later. Good long-range planning will minimize such instances. The long-range plan is not a static document. It is the responsibility of the owner to periodically update it. Assistance of professional planners should be sought in the original preparation and formal updating of the plan.

It is the responsibility of the owner to oversee financing for the project. The hospital administator must approach the Board of Trustees or an administrative agency for the release of available funds or for generating funds. One of the privileges of ownership is paying for the operation, maintenance, growth, or reconstruction of what one owns. The laboratory is no exception. The Board or the owning entity has to arrange the financing for the laboratory project. The Board has a number of options in arranging for financing (see also chapter 11):

- *Use presently available funds*
- *Borrow against future earnings*
- *Initiate a community fund drive*
- *Lobby for budget (governmental institutions)*
- *Sell bonds*
- *Raise taxes (public institutions)*

As the owner, the pathologist or administrator has the ultimate responsibility for the project oversight. If the Board appoints a building committee, the oversight will be shared. The task of project oversight or scheduling may not necessarily be as difficult as it sounds. A responsible and experienced architect will endeavor to keep both the design and construction phases smooth.

The role of owner requires considerable skill in arbitration and mediation. The owner has to arbitrate among various contending sections for space, facilities, project phasing, and project priorities. The word arbitration is used here in an informal sense. Formal arbitration rarely is needed. In such cases the owner may not be the arbitrator but is a party to arbitration. Formal arbitration can be invoked in the event of serious disputes between the owner and the architect or between the institution and the contractor. The Board has a similar responsibility in managing and resolving conflicts. The additional authority that the Board has is to resolve the conflicts between the administrator and other parties within the institution. Furthermore, the Board will be involved in all external litigations involving the institution.

The administrator or owner should function as liaison with the Board, community, and various agencies where applicable. It is the responsibility of the administrator to seek authorization for the laboratory project and to keep the Board and others advised at significant points. A hospital may have a public relations section, but the administrator is still the principal representative of the hospital to the community.

If consultant selection is for the laboratory project only, a hospital administrator should ask the pathologist to be involved. If the consultant is to be selected for the hospital as a whole, then several members of the medical staff, including the pathologist, may be asked to be involved. The administrator and/or the Board would make the final decision. The Board has the final say in engaging consultants and architects. For smaller projects, the Board may authorize the administrator to engage the consultant and the architect. For larger projects, the members of the Board may want to interview a number of prospective consultants and architects and make the final decision.

Others Involved in the Planning and Design Process

Laboratory Consultant

Either the planner or the architect, or both, may be experienced and knowledgeable about laboratory planning and equipment. However, this is not always the case. The services of a laboratory consultant may be useful. The laboratory consultant generally has evolved from the ranks of pathologists, architects, and planners. The laboratory consultant should assist the owner, pathologist, and architect with detailed knowledge of laboratory equipment and the functional intricacies of each section of the laboratory.

" . . . The laboratory consultant generally has evolved from the ranks of pathologists, architects, and planners. "

17

Review Agencies

A number of review agencies may be involved in a laboratory project. The larger the project, the greater the probability that agencies will be involved. There are generally four areas in which review agencies may involve themselves in a laboratory project:

- *Plan and project review and approval (Certificate of Need)*
- *Conformance with regulations*
- *Accreditation*
- *Community input*

Many projects over a certain dollar value will require a Certificate of Need from the health planning agency having jurisdiction over that state. A second level of approval usually will be needed from the state health planning agency which may also review the plans at certain stages. Most hospitals get some patient care funds from the federal government, therefore necessitating compliance with federal regulations.

In addition to complying with the planning guidelines and regulations of these agencies, the project has to conform with regulations on local zoning, building, fire safety, life safety, and OSHA. The architect is knowledgeable about building codes and should ensure they are complied with. Occasionally, a project is initiated when an existing building deteriorates to the point of failing to meet current building codes. When the hospital undertakes a project for a part of the facility, such as the laboratory, the agencies may require that the total facility be improved to meet current codes.

Accreditation is important for institutions. It indicates the institution meets the standards set by the accrediting agency. The Joint Commission on Accreditation of Hospitals (JCAH) inspects the premises, reviews the operational procedures, and issues the accreditation certificate if the institution meets the required criteria. Alternatively, the laboratory may desire accreditation by the College of American Pathologists, which is accepted by the JCAH in lieu of its own accreditation program. Deficiencies pointed out in accreditation reports may be included for correction in the design project.

At the local and state levels, the agency may provide a mechanism for community input. Input may be supportive or nonsupportive of the project. A competitive community group may view the project as a threat and attempt to stop the project. Fortunately, strong opposition such as this is usually the exception rather than the rule. Astute Board members and administrators will be able to sense the opposition before the project is too far advanced.

Medical Staff

The medical staff is the client of the laboratory. The medical staff members order the tests to be performed for the patients. These physicians, who use the test results, have a vested interest in getting accurate test results within a reasonable time. This could be considered the primary mission of any laboratory. The medical staff may have suggestions for services desired from the laboratory. Nurses and other hospital staff sometimes have good suggestions to improve the working relationship between the laboratory and other sections. The renovation or reconstruction project for the laboratory provides a wonderful opportunity for incorporating many ideas for improvement. Areas of potential improvement may include the following:

- *Facilities for performing new tests, or doing some tests faster or more accurately, may be incorporated into the project.*
- *Location of the laboratory in proper functional relationship to the ER, surgery, and outpatient sections. If the project offers the opportunity for a better location, this should be pursued.*
- *Prompt test results reporting is important to efficient health care delivery. Often there is an inordinate delay between completion of the test and reporting of the results. A computerized information system can improve reporting considerably.*

There is concern in the health care community that too many tests are being ordered and too many of these are marked "STAT." Some medical schools are now offering courses on appropriate use of the laboratory with a view toward decreasing the number of tests ordered. With advanced equipment, routine tests can be done quickly. If reliable test results can be made available on time, abuse of STAT will be reduced. This is a point well worth addressing in any laboratory project.

Equipment Planners

The pathologist should be familiar with equipment alternatives and be able to select the optimum equipment for the specific laboratory. If the pathologist is not totally familiar with various alternative equipment available, he may seek the help of a laboratory equipment planner. The architect should acquire installation and utility requirement information from the equipment planner, pathologist, or manufacturer. Greater knowledge of the desired laboratory instruments and equipment at an early stage of design will give the architect more flexibility in placing the equipment. The development of automated analyzers, computerization of the laboratory, and the future introduction of robotics have profound impact on laboratory planning.

Cost Estimator (Quantity Surveyor)

At each design phase, the architect or other specialist will provide an estimate of probable construction cost. It is important for the owner to understand that the probable construction cost provided by the architect is not a commitment. The commitment to construct the facility for a certain price is made by the contractor, not by the architect. In the British Commonwealth countries, quantity surveyors prepare detailed estimates based on the architect's drawings. This profession has started filtering into the United States. Some architects in the United States use quantity surveyors to prepare the estimate of probable construction cost.

THE LABORATORY PLANNING AND DESIGN PROCESS IN HISTORICAL PERSPECTIVE 4

LABORATORY PLANNING AND DESIGN HAS EVOLVED in recent years into a complex process requiring a team approach and considerable effort in data base collection and programming. In past years the planning process involved primarily the pathologist, chief technologist, and architect. Often, none of these individuals was experienced in the design process of laboratories. These efforts frequently resulted in laboratories that looked uncomfortably similar to student laboratories. In addition, the laboratory may not have fit functionally into the overall mission of the institution or setting it served. The flexibility of these laboratories for future expansion and adaptation to new and emerging technologies was limited.

Virtually nothing was published on the process of laboratory planning and design before the end of World War II. It was not until the late 1940s and early 1950s that articles and books were published presenting methods for the planning and design of laboratories. One of the earliest publications was developed by the Division of Hospital Facilities of the United States Public Health Service. This and similar publications presented laboratory design by printing examples of various laboratory plans that were constructed in hospitals. There was little or no discussion regarding the process to program, plan, and design a laboratory. No mention was made of the applications of utilization rates, test volumes, types of health care programs, mechanical/electrical services needs, personnel, etc., and the impact of these factors on laboratory requirements.

In 1960 Dr. Arthur E. Rappaport produced the *Manual for Laboratory Planning and Design*. This manual was published by the College of American Pathologists and was the result of much input from many pathologists and others interested in the planning process. It was the first serious attempt to develop a programming and planning methodology for clinical laboratories. Although much of the data in this manual is somewhat obsolete by contemporary facilities' standards, it is still considered the forerunner in the effort to establish principles for programming and planning of clinical laboratories.

Subsequent to Dr. Rappaport's efforts, other manuals were published presenting different approaches for planning clinical laboratories. Many of these publications used the relationship of laboratory area (gross square feet) to the number of beds in the institution. This gross-square-foot-per-bed "factor" became so popular as the basis for planning medical laboratories that many states incorporated these factors into the rules and regulations that were established relative to planning hospitals under the many state and federal programs developed in the 1950s and 1960s.

Other individuals with extensive experience in the health care field and with concern for developing a planning process, began to publish. E. Todd Wheeler, FAIA, an architect, published *Hospital Design and Function* in 1964. This textbook was among the first to apply mathematical and statistical models in planning the functions and activities of a hospital including laboratories. It is still considered a useful reference. Such publications recognized that a number of factors (other than number of beds), including the type and number of tests, operational goals and objectives, community needs and resources, should determine the ultimate size and configuration of the laboratory facility.

The Laboratory Workload Recording Method, originally developed in Canada and later modified by the College of American Pathologists, is used throughout Canada and by many laboratories in the United States. It is one of the useful tools in determining area or square-foot requirements for a laboratory and also can produce a reliable measure for determining the number of laboratory personnel required. The CAP *Workload Recording Manual* is now updated annually.

The CAP *Manual for Laboratory Planning and Design* was updated in 1977. Many changes in the health care delivery system, new government regulations, advances in medical technology, and biomedical testing and analysis equipment, signaled the need for a more scientific approach to laboratory planning and design. Architectural, mechanical, and electrical engineering requirements also became more complex. This manual update was presented as a checklist to assist in the process. The manual presented examples of laboratories that were considered by their user as functional and well designed. Charts were included that show relationships among hospitals relative to laboratory space allocation, teaching programs, number of staff, number of procedures, automation, gross square feet, net square feet, inpatient and outpatient load, square feet per person, and linear feet of work counter per person.

The American Institute of Architects, through its Subcommittee on Programming and Design of the Committee on Architecture for Health, has recently developed a guideline entitled *Determining Hospital Space Requirements*. This publication presents a planning methodology that stresses functional requirements as the basis for planning and design of hospital facilities including laboratories.

These most recent publications clearly recognize that the traditional gross-square-foot-per-bed factor is not valid as a planning method for clinical laboratories, or for any other hospital function. Planning consultants and other professionals in the field no longer recommend or use these traditional planning factors. To determine the square-foot requirements, layout, and interior design, emphasis is placed on analysis of service use including numbers of tests performed, types of tests to be performed, hospital and community served, health care programs, etc.

FUTURE PERSPECTIVES 5

EVER SINCE THE FIRST SHELTER built by humans, slow evolutionary changes have taken place in construction methods. Only two developments in the history of construction can be described as quantum leaps and sea changes.

1. *The ability to construct multistoried buildings.*
2. *The ability to control interior environment (i.e., heating, ventilation, air-conditioning, and light).*

No such quantum leap is expected in the near future. Development of construction technology in space and on the moon may provide us with new knowledge that can be applied to construction methods on earth.

On a secondary level, a continuous stream of changes and improvements occur, some of which will affect laboratory construction in the future.

Changes in Construction and Design Methods

Moveable Partitions

Because of the inherent flexibility of moveable partitions, they have become popular in the laboratory. Moveable partitions still do not offer satisfactory acoustic privacy, and some improvements may be expected in the future. With the exception of spaces posing microbiological hazards, it will be possible to define all other spaces in the laboratory with moveable partitions.

Changing Utility Requirements

The clinical laboratory has evolved into a high-technology industry. Requirements for fuel gas have given way to requirements for data and voice communication lines. Diminishing dependence of the laboratory on fixed and wet utilities will have a significant impact on the layout of the laboratory.

Carpet Tiles and Flat Cables

This is a recent development that responds directly to the changing utility requirements. Data, power, and communication lines are incorporated into flat cables laid on the floor. Then the floor is covered with carpet tiles instead of broadloom. Access to data, power, and communication lines is immediately available just by lifting one carpet tile. The moveable partitions can be energized by tying into the flat cable system.

Modular, Moveable, Multifunction Casework

During the past decade, a great deal of attention has been given to laboratory casework. The development of such systems as the Herman Miller Action Office and Health/Science co/struc component systems has ushered in a new era of work stations to the laboratory. Many other companies offer excellent competitive products. Further development and refinement in this area will continue to take place. Components for CRT, printer, and EDP storage are available now.

Moveable, Flexible, Utility Connections

While flat cables or other as yet unknown devices will take care of power, communication, and data lines, there will still be the need for some wet lines for water, and possibly lines for gas and vacuum. With the development of improved rubber, plastic, nylon, and PVC pipes, these utility lines could be tapped from a ceiling grid and wastelines connected to a floor grid. This will virtually eliminate the utility core that has dominated the laboratory design for so long.

Prefabricated Building Systems

Prefabricated buildings have not been successful in the United States. The huge investment in the prefabrication factory requires a large market for identical or similar components. Buildings in the United States are too diverse and customized for prefabricated building components. Further development of robotics can change this. Robots can produce custom items almost at the same speed as standard items. The difference between a mechanical machine and a robot (an intelligent electronic machine with mechanical parts) is that a mechanical machine can do routine things quickly, while a robot can do nonroutine

> *" . . . Diminishing dependence of the laboratory on fixed and wet utilities will have a significant impact on the layout of the laboratory. "*

26

things quickly. As the use of robots in the United States increases, so will the use of prefabricated building components.

Solar Energy

Architects are beginning to relearn that the inherent design of the building based on basic age-old principles is more effective than applied contraptions. First of all, the building has to be oriented correctly (correct orientation depends on a number of environmental and geographic factors such as latitude, contours, etc.). Secondly, a simple sunshade that stops the sun in the summer but lets the sun in during the winter, can be just as effective as expensive and complicated trombe walls and other building modifications.

New Systems of Fire Suppression

Water is an effective fire suppressant. However, the damage caused by water deluge often is not less than property damage caused by fire. Also, water is not a good neutralizer of smoke. Water deluge in an intensive care unit can be dangerous.

New development in fire and smoke suppression systems has progressed. Inert chemicals instead of water are released in order to suppress smoke and fire. More improvement in this area is necessary and undoubtedly will occur.

Communication

Communications is, and is going to remain, a dynamic field during the coming decade. It may not be long before inhouse teleconferencing is available at every major institution. Improved communications within hospitals will drastically reduce the turnaround time for test results. Test results will be made available to the physician ordering the test immediately after the test is done. Currently, this process takes hours in most institutions. There will be greater electronic control of the laboratory's environment. Not just temperature and humidity, but information on radiation and microbiological levels will become more routine and public.

Heat Recovery Systems

Heat recovery systems are methods of energy conservation. Two parallel methods of heat recovery exist. One is to recycle heat generated by lights, equipment, and people within the building. The other is to seal the building tightly and recover heat from the air being exhausted.

Unfortunately, the tightly sealed building has posed serious health hazards. A building that does not leak has little margin for error in case of air contamination. An example is the occurrence of Legionnaire's Disease in a hotel in Philadelphia. It has now been established that Legionnaire's Disease is a building-contamination-generated disease. Laboratory designers need to be especially sensitive to this issue.

How to resolve the conflicting requirements of energy conservation and building hygiene is going to be a topic of discussion and research for the next several years.

Changes in the Health Care Delivery System

The future laboratory will be heavily influenced by technological advances as indicated previously. In addition, the health care delivery system is currently in a period of change with great impact from federal and state governments, by economic limits, and by industry as well as the general population. At the time of this writing the final outcome can only be considered a guestimate, but certain trends appear evident. These trends will affect the types of laboratories that will be functioning in the next decade, as well as their location and their type of service commitments.

The capping mechanism as reflected in the 1983 Medicare revisions are now evident to all of us. This has been an interim mechanism awaiting development of a more comprehensive control of medical services in general. The direction of the long-term goal appears to be that of a competitive bidding type of delivery system which will certainly affect type, size, and quality of laboratory functions. One can easily visualize the limited on-site laboratory services in an acute type of situation for many hospitals with the bulk of the general laboratory testing being done at an off-site facility under the competitive bidding type of arrangement. Obviously, during this transition period many hospitals will maintain on-site full service laboratories, but one should be aware of the impact of the change in delivery systems when redesigning or modifying existing laboratory facilities.

There is also the suggestion that federal control will be less prominent in the future with much of the control of health care delivery systems being relegated to the state level. This is obvious in many locations at the time of this writing and will be expected to expand during the remainder of this decade. With the advent of the DRG concept, as well as the competitive bidding concept alluded to, one can anticipate a decrease in volume of testing in many areas and long-range planning should reflect these anticipated changes. In addition, the hospital will become primarily an acute care facility with much of the medical care being provided in outpatient and physician office facilities. Again, this will impact on the laboratory volume and general needs.

The concept of profit versus nonprofit hospital systems appears to be well established, and it is anticipated that there will be growth in both areas, with development of large multihospital systems inevitable in order to take advantage of the large scale for control of economic resources. Smaller laboratories will diminish and be replaced by the larger regionalized or multisystems laboratories. In the future, laboratories will be hospital-based, or regionally related, or totally free of any hospital relationship or function. All of these laboratories will be competitive with one another.

As mentioned previously, the health care industry is in a period of great change. It is being impacted by many forces including federal regulatory and legislative changes, industrial coalitions, and the general public. The overall result is expected to be a total reduction in dollars spent for medical services. The effect on the laboratory segment is not totally clear, but certain trends seem to be emerging. Some studies suggest that if the ancillary services of a hospital are reduced by less than 10 percent, there is no significant cost savings. Therefore, one can anticipate a greater reduction in this area as time passes. Networking, shared services, and multinational laboratories will become the primary mode of laboratory services.

" . . . Design and function then become a feature of the various forces which will affect the delivery of laboratory medicine."

Design and function then become a feature of these various forces which will affect the delivery of laboratory medicine. Hospitals may evolve into efficient acute care laboratories with the bulk of testing being done offsite at a regional or a network type of facility. One may anticipate that the volume of testing per patient will be diminished, but the possibility of an increase in the number of newly developed tests may be anticipated in certain areas.

The concept of bedside testing is being considered seriously by industry. For example, this could supplement or replace the acute care laboratory, as envisioned currently, with the acute care moving to the bedside for specific acute testing with the bulk of laboratory services being provided again in an outside facility. The evolution of this change in the delivery system in the laboratory will certainly be affected by modes of communication and transportation of the specimens to effect reasonable turnaround times. Many other forces will impact on evolving medical services and in designing the laboratory for future use. These variable forces, which will affect the type of laboratory and delivery system involved, should be considered.

The current trend in the health care delivery system affecting hospitals is that of the creation of multiple hospital systems. This appears to be necessary for efficient operation and management of resources and finances as the various federal regulations impact on hospital delivery systems. Also, there appears to be a trend from nonprofit to the for-profit type of hospital operation. This is seen in the absorption of many of the smaller hospitals by for-profit, multinational systems. These changes also will affect the design and function of the inhospital laboratory. Laboratory services also will be seen, as we have indicated earlier, in the regional or networking type of large, multispatial laboratories. Additionally, one must consider the evolution of small laboratory testing within the larger, multiphysician type of complexes.

Changes in the Laboratory Field

Technology

Continued changes can be expected in the future of health care generally and in the laboratory field specifically. Although details cannot be predicted with certainty, various trends seem likely at this time. Technology will continue to grow, with development of new tests, increased automation and cybernetics, instrument miniaturization, and computerization. Along with this, certain new trends in technology will include therapeutic drug monitoring, immunofluorescent assays (in tissue studies, microbiology, and immunology), radioimmunoassays (RIA), ELISA techniques, use of cell markers in oncologic hematology and pathology, immunoperoxidase staining techniques, chromosome analysis, lymphocyte typing, electron microscopy, and magnetic resonance spectroscopy. Noninvasive techniques (such as blood gases) will be more common. Pheresis services will include plasmapheresis and granulocyte transfusions. Pathologists probably will offer new consultation services, often with computer-generated data and correlations. New instrument developments with miniaturization and freestanding features will alter laboratory space requirements and design.

Space, Workload, and Test Mix

Future trends toward laboratory expansion can be expected. However, there are indications that this trend for increasing space requirements may be offset considerably and possibly reversed. A multitude of factors could lead to this reversal. These include the impact of the regulatory agencies, the economic pressures on government and private health insurers to reduce expenditures, the trend to development of independent freestanding facilities, and cost-containment measures such as the DRG prospective payment system. Competition by commercial laboratories, regional specialty laboratory systems, HMOs, hospital mergers, and integrated health delivery systems are other factors. Workload volume will probably level off because of proposed rate review and cost-control commissions, tendency towards institution specialization, and bedside testing. The test mix will be altered by a tendency toward fewer profiles and more organ panels and discrete tests.

Personnel

Personnel changes can be expected. With increased automation and computerization, the need for skilled medical technologists may be decreased for routine work. However, they will be needed in supervisory roles and for evaluation and development of new methodologies, techniques, and new equipment. All these factors will probably result in more routine work performed by less-skilled people, with decrease in the need for medical technologists. As a result of these and other factors, good laboratory design planning becomes increasingly more important. The development of information service needs within the laboratory will require employment of personnel with special skills, e.g., information service specialists.

Adaptation to Change

If future changes are not anticipated and flexibility has not been incorporated into the design, adaptation to future and unpredictable needs will be restricted. For example, there may not be access for new and larger technical instruments if the corridors and doors to individual laboratories are too small. As the usage of autologous blood increases in the face of risks from heterologous blood donors, as in the AIDS problem, space must be available for drawing blood from donors and storage of the blood. Problems may occur if flexible space is not available for changes from noncomputerized to computerized laboratory systems and to accommodate for shifts in workload requiring more space in one department and less in another.

Provisions should be made for increased interpretive reporting with computer assistance, use of microcomputers in the various offices and work areas of the laboratory, and transmission of reports directly to the physician's office. Consideration should be given to the need for shielded electric lines for future needs.

Thus, trying to determine projected laboratory growth rate will be difficult at best, augmenting the need for flexible plans. These plans should include properly located soft space for later conversion, if and when necessary. Also, the laboratory location and design should allow areas for contiguous expansion. In all this planning, the cost of present construction must be balanced against that of future construction.

Robotics in the Laboratory

Karel Capek, a Czechoslovakian playwright, coined the word "robot" in a play he wrote in 1920. At that time, it was sheer fantasy. Today, robots are becoming useful tools in our industrial community and clinical laboratories throughout the country.

Several decades ago, the noted science fiction writer, Isaac Asimov, wrote the story *I, Robot*. In the story he developed the *Three Laws of Robotics*. It is of interest to list them here because of the enormous potential robots will have, not only in an industrial setting, but in society as well.

1. *A robot may not injure a human being or, through inaction, allow a human being to come to harm.*

2. *A robot must obey the orders given it by human beings, except where such orders would conflict with the first law.*

3. *A robot must protect its own existence, as long as such protection does not conflict with the first or second law.*

Robots as machines have been with us for many years. However, it was not until the development of microcomputers that robotics have taken a new evolutionary direction to becoming sophisticated adjuncts to many industrial processes.

Their introduction into the laboratory began with simple machines,

> **"** . . . *Trying to determine projected laboratory growth rate will be difficult at best, augmenting the need for flexible plans.* **"**

32

such as centrifuges and mixers, etc. More recently, robots are being perfected with sensitive touch, position sensors, vision capabilities, and locomotion. Some robots are even being equipped with adaptive intelligence.

Presently, most of the robots being developed for industrial and laboratory use are designed to do repetitive kinds of tasks such as mixing, sorting, and specimen preparation. Other robots are being developed to work in hazardous types of environments.

For many years, in nuclear physics laboratories, automated manipulators were developed so that hazardous materials could be handled by personnel from behind a protective shield. These manipulators are a direct result of a science fiction story that was written originally in the 1920s. The story depicted the need for humans to be able to handle hazardous materials while being protected behind a screen or shield. These manipulators described by the author were nicknamed "Elmers." This name has remained and the robot manipulators that are used in physics laboratories are called Elmers in honor of this author.

The industry that is producing robots is expanding rapidly each year. It has been projected that there will be several hundred thousand robots of different types in American industry and laboratories by the year 1990.

At present, several companies manufacture robots for clinical laboratory application. One such company has developed robots to remove interferences and contaminants from samples, modify the sample to enhance detection, then convert it to the appropriate form for instrumental analysis. This process is accomplished by the robot transferring vials and tubes from sample racks to a variety of preparation stations located within its reach. This reach varies within the capabilities of the particular machine. Another "intelligent" special purpose robot uses standard microliter syringes to transfer samples, reagents, and standards.

It is conceivable that within the next several years as the technology evolves, robots will be developed to perform more and more complicated tasks that are currently performed by human laboratory technicians. The implication is not that laboratory technicians will become obsolete, but that robots will be devised to accomplish the more routine tasks that are essentially repetitious. Thus, such machines can improve the level of accuracy, and permit technicians and staff to perform the more complicated procedures. The laboratory of the future may perform all routine tests by using robots, except those of a special nature.

> *" . . . Robots will be developed to perform more and more complicated tasks that are currently performed by human laboratory technicians."*

Many automated analyzers now in use can be considered robots. Such machines, when they were first developed, were large and bulky. Presently, the newer generation machines are more complicated, smaller, and have become more reliable through the use of microelectronics and microprocessor circuitry.

Robots are available to do automatic filtrations. Others can be set up for sample conditioning stations providing vortex mixing and temperature and atmosphere control. Possible future robot stations will include a homogenizer station, centrifuge, an electronic balance, injectors for high performance liquid chromatographs, sample introduction for colorimeters, and spectrophotometers. The list of procedures that robots can perform grows daily.

How will this affect the programming, planning, and design of laboratories? This is a difficult question to answer at this time. However, with the robots and other automated machines that are available, those involved in the planning process must take into account the special requirements for such machines. These requirements may involve special mechanical or electrical services, special structural requirements, special service/maintenance requirements, specially trained personnel, etc.

Certainly, education programs for laboratory technicians should be modified to expose this new technology to the students. Computer technology is already an integrated system within the laboratory administration and operation. The robot will become another addition to the computer systems technology in the laboratory. The limit to which robots can be used in a laboratory will be limited to the technology capability and imagination of the individuals involved.

The application of automation and robotics in the laboratory must not be overlooked. Pathologists, architects, planners, and others involved in the process of developing the plan for a laboratory must include this new technology in the planning process. These specialized machines require a different type of trained technician and a different physical environment as well. It is unlikely that computers and robots will eliminate any particular job or task that is currently done by human technicians. However, robots will modify the tasks that have been traditionally performed by human technicians. Also, it is clear that the introduction of the automated equipment in the laboratories will slow down the rate of increase in personnel and have a moderating impact on space requirements over any given period of time.

The best advice that can be offered regarding automation, computers, and robotics is that persons involved in the programming and planning of laboratories should investigate this area carefully and integrate the capabilities of these machines into the programming and planning methodology that is presented in this manual.

GRAPHIC TOOLS OF THE PLANNING AND DESIGN PROCESS 6

HE ARCHITECT'S LANGUAGE IS THE DRAWING. It serves two important purposes: first, to act as a tool for the architect in developing a design concept; and second, to communicate the architectural design to others.

The architect uses drawings to explore the design problem and develop the solution. On most projects, the architect functions as a member of a team composed of people from various disciplines with diverse skills. These disciplines include architecture, planning, structural engineering, mechanical engineering, civil engineering, cost estimating, etc. Drawings serve as a common basis of communication.

As a communication device, the drawing explains the design to others. It is a way of presenting the proposed building clearly, and is not an end in itself.

66 ... The architect's language is the drawing. 99

The architectural design process consists of a number of phases. The style and technique of the drawing changes from phase to phase. Initially, the drawing may be loose and sketchy, reflecting the early exploration in the conceptual design phase. As the design solution becomes more clearly defined, the drawings become more detailed and refined.

A brief description of various phases of architectural design and the use and format of drawings in each phase follows. The emphasis is on the progression of complexity in the drawings. A much more detailed discussion of each of the design phases is included in chapters 7, 12, 15, and 17 and complete definitions are included in the glossary.

An example of the planning and design of a hematology section is shown. The materials are by no means comprehensive, but an example of the range and variety of documents which both the user and designer must be familiar with.

Conceptual Ideas—The Program Phase

The architectural space program numerically defines the space requirements of a project in a systematic manner. The program is not part of the architectural design; it precedes the design. The program defines the architectural problem that architectural design must solve.

Drawings are not necessarily a formal part of the program phase, but they can be helpful. For example, drawings that show sizes of key rooms and their furniture layout make abstract numbers more understandable to the client and user.

Preparation of the architectural space program usually is not part of the architect's basic services. The architect may prepare the program as an additional service. Often, the program is written by a consultant, the owner's planning staff, or a separate architect planner (Fig. 6.1).

Bubble, Block, and Schematic Drawings—The Schematic Design Phase

Schematic design is the first phase of the architectural design process. Intensive interaction between the architect and owner/users takes place during this phase. This is when the basic concept, the relationship among spaces, and the scope and size of the project are determined. The drawings have to be most intelligible to the owner and users in this phase.

Schematic design begins with conceptual design. A number of alternative concepts for organizing the laboratory space is developed. Simple bubble diagrams explain relationships.

A bubble diagram is a technique used to establish the relationship among spaces. A bubble, which is usually a freehand-drawn circle, represents a space. The relationship between a number of spaces can be explored quickly without concern about the scale, size, and other constraints.

Using the bubble diagram technique, the architect can quickly test a hierarchy of relationships. For example, if the architect is dealing with a hospital laboratory, the first series of bubble diagrams will be used to explore the relationship between the laboratory and other sections of the hospital, such as radiology, surgery, emergency, supply processing and distribution, and inpatient areas.

The second series of bubble diagrams explores the relationship among the various sections within the laboratory, such as accession, chemistry, coagulation, hematology, offices, etc. (Figs. 6.2 and 6.3). The third series of bubble diagrams explore the relationship among the spaces within each of these sections (Fig. 6.4).

> **"** . . . *As the design solution becomes more clearly defined, the drawings become more detailed and refined.* **"**

38

structural system. These are typically single-line sketches, meaning that the wall thicknesses will not be accurately represented but merely shown as a single line. With this first set of sketches, the objective is to translate the functional relationships specified in the block diagrams into a scale drawing. The space allocation program in specifying square footage area desired for the function will, in turn, be converted into representations of the square footage area.

In developing the initial schematic sketches, block areas and rooms drawn to scale are quickly laid out and composed in a series of alternative relationships. While the objective is to achieve a schematic design that most closely represents the nonscale blocks and bubble diagrams, it quickly becomes apparent that by dealing with the square-foot requirements specified in the space allocation program, conflicts arise. The root of these conflicts is the inability to achieve all the ideal functional relationships specified in the bubble diagram due to the conflicts of scale and area which we are now imposing on the design. By

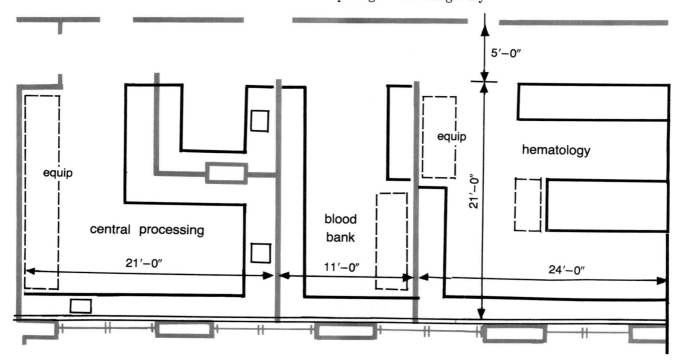

Fig. 6.6

An initial schematic plan showing more detail than in the block diagram. To illustrate how problems may be solved at this stage, note that a CRT station is drawn at the end of a counter in hematology. The hematology supervisor questions whether this space is adequate. See the next figure.

constructing a number of layouts which can be compared to the functional relationships expressed in the earlier bubble diagrams and block drawings, an analysis is made of the most appropriate compromise if one is necessary.

Working from a gross scale to a detailed scale is generally the most expeditious and effective means of proceeding during schematic design. The alternative is to work from the most detailed level of a particular work station and room up to the gross layout for the entire section or building. Obviously, it is important that the designer keep in mind the end product when doing the gross layout while not being bogged down by an inability to work out every detail on the first sketch. It is preferable to work out the overall problems or relationships, shapes, proportions of spaces, and integration with other building systems at this early sketch stage (Fig. 6.7). Through the evolution of the schematic designs, more detail is added until the drawings are responsive to all the requirements developed during the earlier phases (Fig. 6.8).

Laboratory equipment plays an important role not only in the use of the space, but also in the formation and definition of space as well. Therefore, layout of casework and laboratory equipment, often postponed to the design development phase, should be started in the schematic design phase. This allows the pathologist and technologist to provide input on equipment information at an early stage. The architect tests the spaces for efficiency in laying out the equipment and considers utility, communication, and power requirements of the laboratory (Fig. 6.9).

Architectural symbols are relatively standardized but not rigidly so. The owner/user should understand all architectural symbols used beginning in the schematic design phase (Table 6.1).

Several of the most definitive references for symbols and standards are contained in the following publications:

Packard RT, ed (AIA): *Architectural graphic standards*, ed 7. New York, John Wiley and Sons, 1981.

Callender, JH (ed): *Time-saver standards for architectural design data*, ed 6. New York, McGraw-Hill Co., 1980.

DeChiara J, Callender JH (eds): *Time-saver standards for building types*, ed 4. New York: McGraw Hill Co., 1973.

An excellent reference to assist in understanding working drawings is: McHugh RC: *Working drawing handbook*. New York, Van Nostrand Reinhold, 1983.

> **❝ . . . The layout of casework and laboratory equipment, often postponed to the design development phase, should be started in the schematic design phase. ❞**

44

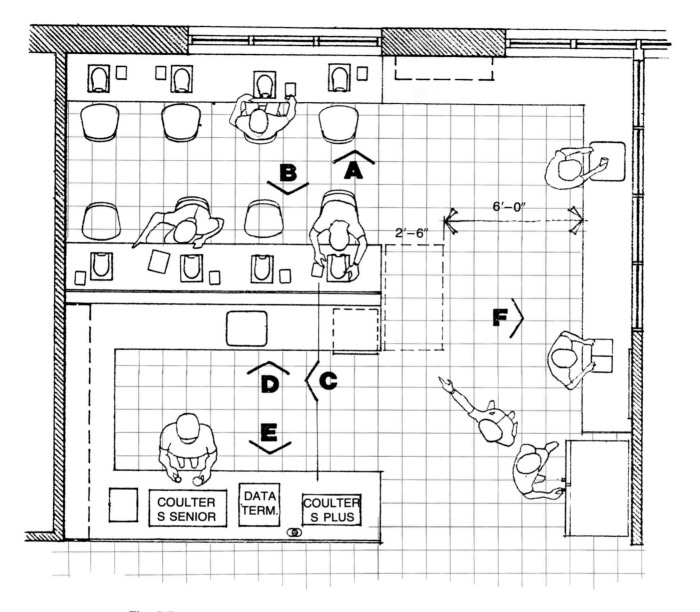

Fig. 6.7

This figure illustrates how specific space problems may be approached. To illustrate more graphically the space relationships in hematology, the designer has produced a scale drawing showing people and equipment. After producing this drawing the supervisor was satisfied there was enough space at the end of the counter for placement of the CRT station. Drawings of this type are not generally part of the schematic drawings.

Hematology Analyzer Work Station

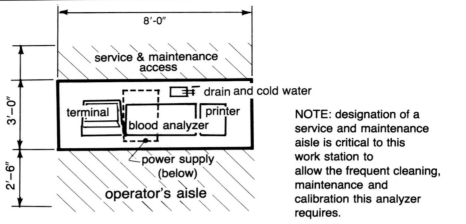

8'-0"

service & maintenance access

3'-0"

2'-6"

drain and cold water

terminal

printer

blood analyzer

power supply (below)

operator's aisle

NOTE: designation of a service and maintenance aisle is critical to this work station to allow the frequent cleaning, maintenance and calibration this analyzer requires.

System Communication Work Station

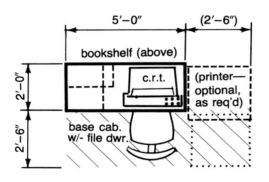

5'-0" (2'-6")

bookshelf (above)

2'-0"

2'-6"

c.r.t.

(printer—optional, as req'd)

base cab. w/- file dwr.

NOTE: this station may be used throughout the lab, it is not customized for hematology

General Laboratory Work Station

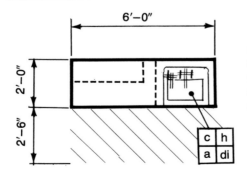

6'-0"

2'-0"

2'-6"

NOTE: a symbol & legend describe service requirements—in this case h = hot; c = cold; di = deionized water; a = acid waste.

c | h
a | di

Fig. 6.8 After the general layout is decided on more attention can be given to specific design problems. Examples of specific work station designs are shown for the hematology area. Drawings of this type are of great help to both the architect and user. These types of drawings are done during the schematic design phase.

46

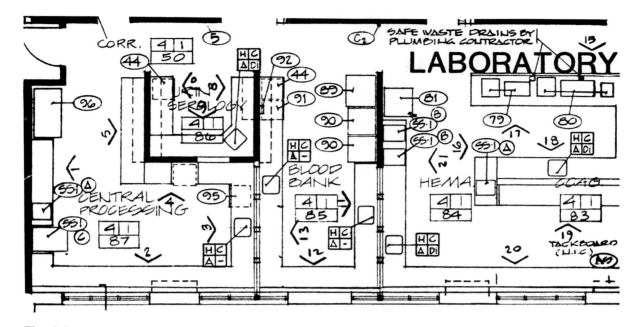

Fig. 6.9

An example of the equipment drawing for the hematology area.

An excellent encyclopedia may be found in: Stein JS, ed (AIA, FCSI): *Construction glossary*. New York, John Wiley and Sons, 1980.

Design Development Documents—The Design Development Phase

Design development is the second phase of the architectural design phase. The building structural system is developed during the design development phase.

After approval of the schematic design by the owner, the architect begins the design development phase. Any changes in the layout from schematic design can be accommodated during the early stage of design development. Later, changes involve a larger number of disciplines such as structural engineers, mechanical engineers, electrical engineers, and others who may be working on the project.

During the design development phase of a laboratory design, the participation of the owner and user is helpful especially in the final selection and placement of laboratory equipment, benchwork, utilities, communication systems, etc. Definition of equipment requirements stated in the schematic design phase should be refined and completed during the design development phase.

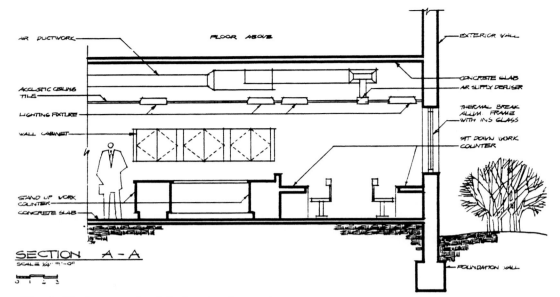

Fig. 6.10 An example of design development.

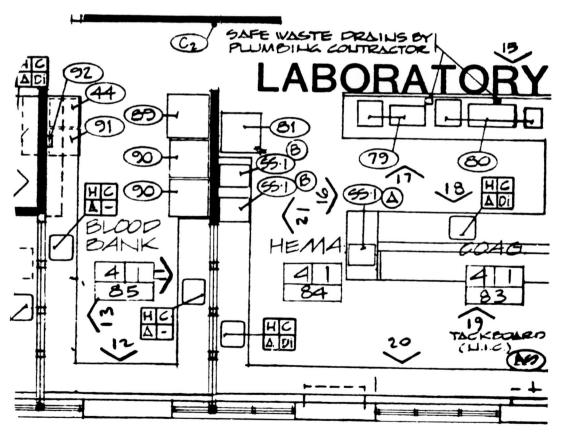

Fig. 6.11 An example of the working drawing for the hematology area.

48

Table 6.1 Table of Common Architectural Symbols

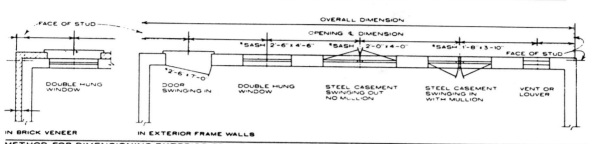

METHOD FOR DIMENSIONING EXTERIOR FRAME WALLS & OPENINGS

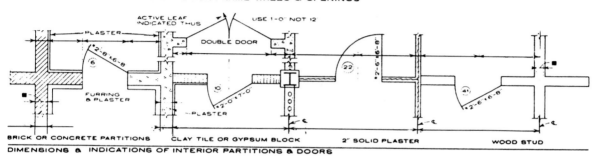

DIMENSIONS & INDICATIONS OF INTERIOR PARTITIONS & DOORS

Walls

MATERIALS

Partitions

Floors

Table 6.1 Table of Common Architectural Symbols *continued*

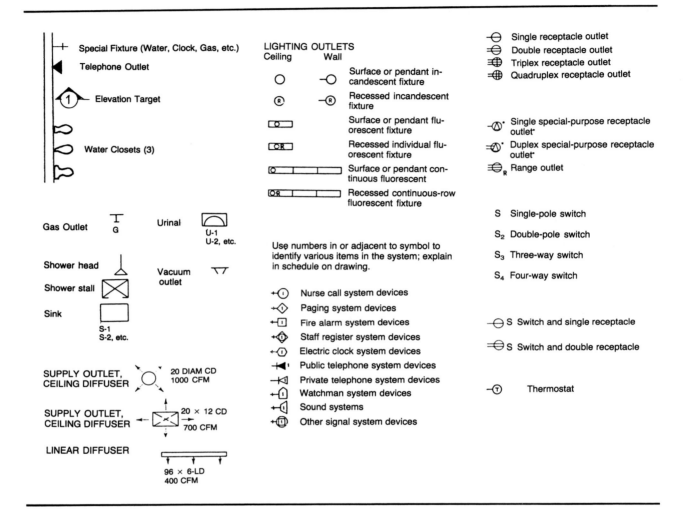

Special Fixture (Water, Clock, Gas, etc.)

Telephone Outlet

Elevation Target

Water Closets (3)

Gas Outlet

Urinal
U-1
U-2, etc.

Shower head

Shower stall

Vacuum outlet

Sink
S-1
S-2, etc.

SUPPLY OUTLET, CEILING DIFFUSER
20 DIAM CD
1000 CFM

SUPPLY OUTLET, CEILING DIFFUSER
20 × 12 CD
700 CFM

LINEAR DIFFUSER
96 × 6-LD
400 CFM

LIGHTING OUTLETS

Ceiling   Wall

Surface or pendant incandescent fixture

Recessed incandescent fixture

Surface or pendant fluorescent fixture

Recessed individual fluorescent fixture

Surface or pendant continuous fluorescent

Recessed continuous-row fluorescent fixture

Use numbers in or adjacent to symbol to identify various items in the system; explain in schedule on drawing.

Nurse call system devices
Paging system devices
Fire alarm system devices
Staff register system devices
Electric clock system devices
Public telephone system devices
Private telephone system devices
Watchman system devices
Sound systems
Other signal system devices

Single receptacle outlet
Double receptacle outlet
Triplex receptacle outlet
Quadruplex receptacle outlet

Single special-purpose receptacle outlet'
Duplex special-purpose receptacle outlet'
Range outlet

S   Single-pole switch
S_2 Double-pole switch
S_3 Three-way switch
S_4 Four-way switch

S Switch and single receptacle
S Switch and double receptacle

Thermostat

Design development drawings may be drawn at ⅛ in = 1 ft or at ¼ in = 1 ft scale with some details shown at a larger scale (Fig. 6.10).

Working Drawings—The Construction Documents Phase

Construction documents show in detail exactly what will be built. Construction documents include working drawings and written specifications. During the bidding phase that follows, construction documents become part of the bid documents. Therefore, construction documents should be easily and completely understood by construction industry people such as contractors and subcontractors (Fig. 6.11).

The construction documents phase is a production process. It is not necessary for the owner and users to be extensively involved in this phase. In a properly sequenced project, all functional decisions would have been made during the schematic design and design development phases.

Working drawings may be drawn at ¼ in = 1 ft scale or other suitable scale depending on the size of the project. Details are drawn at a larger scale.

Bidding and Negotiating Phase

Construction documents prepared by the architect plus any other bidding information generated by the owner comprise the bid documents. The prospective general contractor uses these documents to prepare a price proposal. Usually no new drawings are produced in this phase.

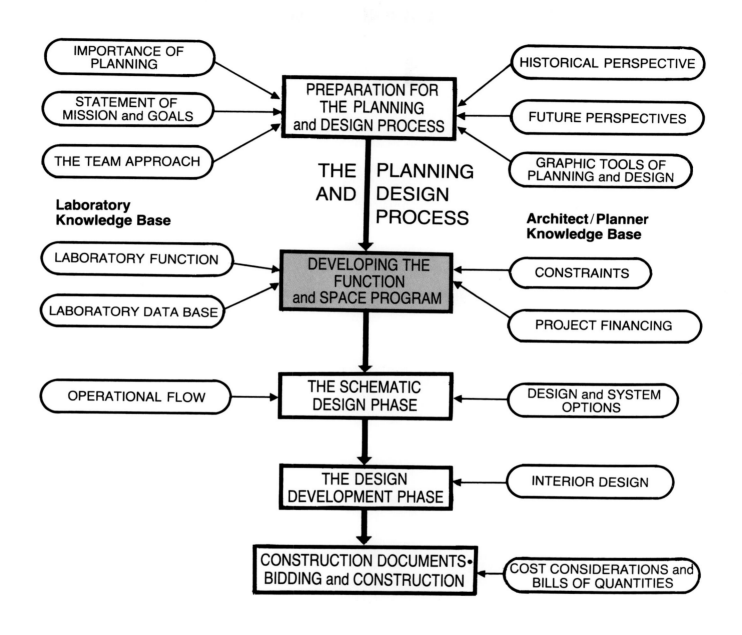

IMPORTANCE OF PLANNING

STATEMENT OF MISSION and GOALS

THE TEAM APPROACH

HISTORICAL PERSPECTIVE

FUTURE PERSPECTIVES

GRAPHIC TOOLS OF PLANNING and DESIGN

PREPARATION FOR THE PLANNING and DESIGN PROCESS

THE PLANNING AND DESIGN PROCESS

Laboratory Knowledge Base

Architect/Planner Knowledge Base

LABORATORY FUNCTION

LABORATORY DATA BASE

DEVELOPING THE FUNCTION and SPACE PROGRAM

CONSTRAINTS

PROJECT FINANCING

OPERATIONAL FLOW

THE SCHEMATIC DESIGN PHASE

DESIGN and SYSTEM OPTIONS

THE DESIGN DEVELOPMENT PHASE

INTERIOR DESIGN

CONSTRUCTION DOCUMENTS• BIDDING and CONSTRUCTION

COST CONSIDERATIONS and BILLS OF QUANTITIES

Part II
DEVELOPING THE FUNCTION AND SPACE PROGRAM

THE FUNCTIONAL AND SPACE PROGRAM 7

GENERALLY, DESIGN PHASES ARE SEQUENTIAL, ideally flowing from one step to the next. However, depending on the size, complexity, and urgency of the proposed project, a number of steps may occur concurrently or be combined with other activities, and in some cases eliminated. The outline presented here is a guide to a design process. An underlying philosophy of this design process is that each laboratory design project is a unique task. Each project must be sufficiently analyzed before and during the design process to ensure the resulting facility is efficient, functional, flexible, pleasant, and safe. The goal of the design process is to achieve these qualities in an expeditious, comprehensive, and accurate manner.

The activities discussed here may precede the formal initiation of design and, in some cases, continue after the principle design tasks are completed. However, if the entire process is understood by the user and the designer, a more successful result can be achieved. This is a process involving people in various roles, all working as a team to achieve an end, i.e., a building which allows the laboratory to perform its work.

Programming

Programming is the process of documenting the requirements of a project with words, numbers, and sometimes sketches. Before programming begins project goals and constraints must be identified and communicated. Typically, a project goal may be as broad as developing a modern and expanded replacement facility to something as specific as expansion of the technician's lounge for accommodating 20 percent more staff.

Constraints or limits which commonly occur include financial budgets, regulatory codes and procedures, and physical constraints such as limited available space due to adjacent buildings, property lines, or other such limits. At this early stage of the project, it is important to be cognizant of constraints. Constraints are to be handled as integral parts of the whole project and not simply

" . . . Programming is the process of documenting the requirement of a project with words, numbers, and sometimes sketches."

avoided. Recognizing them is the first step. They are to be dealt with later in the design process.

Many laboratory planning and design projects occur as independent projects which develop a facility used exclusively by the laboratory on a site dedicated to the laboratory building. Other projects deal with the laboratory as a section in a larger institution, such as a hospital, and include other sections in the institution as well. It is important that a perspective of the laboratory's place in a larger project be maintained. The goals and design solutions developed for the laboratory should be integrated with the larger development process.

A fundamental document which should be developed initially is a functional narrative or program. This may be prepared by the pathologist, planner, or other laboratory personnel. It describes in narrative form the functions and activities which occur in the laboratory. In other words, it describes what the laboratory does and how it works. The functional narrative should be comprehensive, including all sections in the laboratory. It should include discussion of relations within a section as well as with other sections. Types of equipment, services, and general environmental requirements should be mentioned and the various professional, technical, and support personnel described.

During the programming phase, the greatest interaction between user and planner/designer occurs. This is a period of intensive investigation, demonstration, and analysis. The goal of this phase is to quantify the types and sizes of the various components which are necessary in the final design. The tabulation of this data is known as the space allocation program (aka, space allocation, or space analysis).

The space allocation program lists by section, room, and/or space all of the components of the laboratory. Each component is assigned an area in square feet which represents the net area required to accommodate the equipment, furniture, supplies, people, and circulation space. These become the basic building blocks of the final plan, and their accuracy has a great impact on the ultimate success or failure of the project. An area which is too small compromises the activity it is intended to accommodate. However, an area which is too large may cause inefficient circulation and work stations which are too far apart. An even more serious consequence is the negative impact that additional square footage has on the project cost.

The square footage applied to the rooms and areas up to this point are expressed as net square footage. Gross square footage for these areas and for the buildings are estimated by applying conversion factors to the section net totals to account for section walls, general circulation, mechanical and electrical spaces, as well as the building structure and exterior walls. When prepared correctly, this space allocation program closely represents the exact gross area for which the final building will be designed.

Determination of space required for each function and for the areas which support that function is one of the key elements of the programming phase. By understanding the precise nature of the function and flow of the laboratory, an intelligent decision can be made on the specific space required to accommodate its activities. Ideally, every element which affects the performance of the task desired should be accommodated in the determination of space needs. Multiple factors influence this space need. A fundamental criteria is whether the space is to be occupied by people, people and equipment, equipment and supplies, or simply equipment. Each of these situations involves different space needs.

In many respects, the requirements for people who work in the laboratory are similar to those in any other work environment. Namely, people require the space to move about and an environment which allows them to perform their tasks. This influences the height of their work surfaces, the distance needed to reach for implements they require, the amount of movement required in order to access all of the areas involved in completion of their tasks, and numerous other factors. Likewise, equipment has varying requirements as well. These often are just as rigid, or more rigid, than those required to accommodate the people working in the laboratory.

Some of the basic questions which must be answered in determining space needs are as follows:

- *What are the functions of this area?*

- *What is the flow of people and materials in this area?*

- *How many people will be working in this area?*

- *What equipment will be in this area?*

- *What size will the equipment be in this area?*

- *What are the relationships of this area to adjacent areas and therefore, what circulation and access points are required to these adjacent areas?*

" . . . By understanding the precise nature of the function and flow of the laboratory, an intelligent decision can be made on the specific space required to accommodate its activities. "

- *What supplies must be stored in this area?*

- *What are the utilities and services required for tasks in this area?*

- *What furniture and/or casework is required for this area?*

- *Do the functions being planned for occur simultaneously, in sequence, on a scheduled basis, or at random?*

(See chapter 9 on Medical Laboratory Data Base for further explanation of these concepts.)

The answers to these questions and others lead to area determinations in the form of square footage, which can be accumulated into the total space need for this particular area. One approach to space determination is simply to look at individual work stations. The work station is comprised of space to accommodate equipment and apparatus for the task at hand, the technician or technicians involved in performing that task, and the supplies and material required for the performance of the task. A simple example is a secretarial work area. The work area typically may be made up of a 5-ft × 3-ft desk with 3½-ft × 2-ft typing return. The station also has a chair for the secretary and circulation to get to the chair and the desk. Additionally, there also may be other furniture for supplies and files, which also needs circulation for access. Space for all these items is then accumulated and equals the net area required for each work station. A work station in a laboratory can be analyzed in a similar manner. The specific makeup of that space includes decisions such as whether the task will be performed by a person who is standing up or sitting down. The size of the work surface leads directly to a net area for that particular work station. Add to this the area required for a person to sit or stand in front of this work station and space beyond that to circulate in and around this particular work station. In many cases, these circulation areas may be shared with adjacent work stations.

The space needs of equipment go beyond the actual net area to accommodate the so-called footprint of that equipment. For example, an analyzer which is floor-mounted and has dimensions of 3 ft × 4 ft will require more than the 12 net square feet it occupies. Access to one or more sides requires additional space so that panels on the equipment may be swung out, service technicians can comfortably get to that particular area of equipment, and parts can be removed and reinstalled. In addition, the environmental requirements for that particular piece of equipment may require clearances to dissipate heat generated. Again, while these clearances are all vital and necessary, it is not always necessary to dedicate space in a cumulative fashion. Instead, service access and general circulation to each piece of equipment and work station can often over-lap with adjacent pieces and thereby save on the total area required. This is common for pieces of equipment which are used less frequently and generate less traffic. For work stations and equipment which are in constant operation, with high volumes of service, and a large number of people accessing it, circulation may need to be dedicated.

Other miscellaneous factors influence the determination of space size. If the area is to be enclosed by hard partitions, this may influence the overall size of the area. If a door is to swing into the area, this must be recognized as taking up space which cannot be occupied by anything else. Life safety codes, building codes, and worker regulations also may influence the size and layout of the work area by requiring minimum clearances and unobstructed escape routes.

During the programming phase, it is helpful to develop a set of Room Data Sheets (Fig. 7.1). The purpose of these sheets will be to provide information on each specific room and/or area involved in the laboratory. This information ranges from sizes and types of doors in the space, hardware, and other special features on these doors to mechanical services and utilities, special communication requirements, room finishes, casework, and other special conditions. The purpose of the Room Data Sheet is to develop at the onset, a set of quality specifications for each area. It allows the architect to quickly develop, in conjunction with the space allocation program, an accurate representation of the final configuration. It informs all members of the project team the expectations and specific performance anticipated for each area. In addition, it allows for a more accurate cost estimate to be generated at the completion of the initial programming phase. A combination of unit square footage prices, in conjunction with the detailed data provided in the Room Data Sheets, can be used by either the architect or the general contractor to develop an initial price estimate for the project. Obviously, the more accurate the information available, the more accurate the price estimate will be.

The Room Data Sheet often is provided by the planner/programmer. However, it may also be developed by the laboratory representative or the architect.

The first step in translating the space allocation program into a fully developed design is to organize all the components of the space allocation program and graphically illustrate the interrelationships between each component. These types of drawings or sketches are known as relationship drawings (aka, bubble drawings, nonscale block drawings). At this stage, they need not be to scale be-

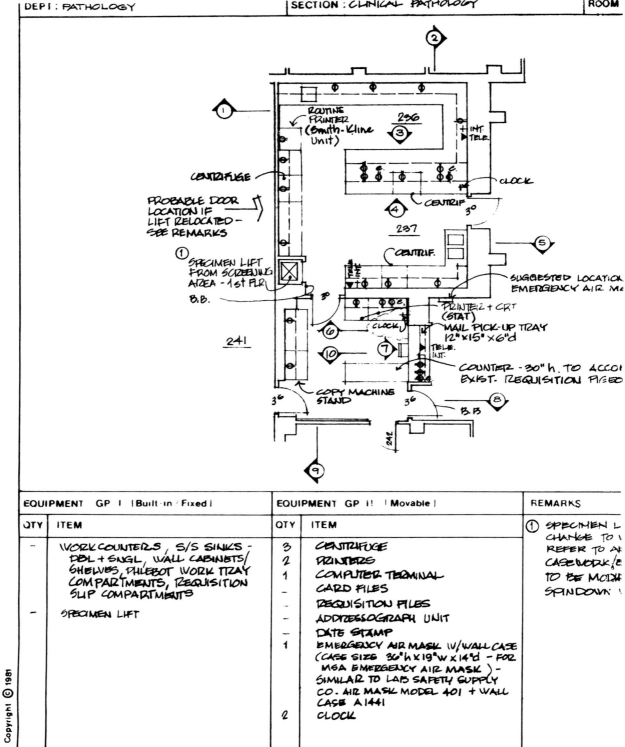

EQUIPMENT GP I (Built-in/Fixed)		EQUIPMENT GP II (Movable)		REMARKS
QTY	ITEM	QTY	ITEM	① SPECIMEN L
–	WORK COUNTERS, S/S SINKS - DBL + SNGL, WALL CABINETS/ SHELVES, PHLEBOT WORK TRAY COMPARTMENTS, REQUISITION SLIP COMPARTMENTS	3	CENTRIFUGE	CHANGE TO
		2	PRINTERS	REFER TO A
		1	COMPUTER TERMINAL	CASEWORK/E
		–	CARD FILES	TO BE MODIF
–	SPECIMEN LIFT	–	REQUISITION FILES	SPINDOWN
		–	ADDRESSOGRAPH UNIT	
		–	DATE STAMP	
		1	EMERGENCY AIR MASK W/ WALL CASE (CASE SIZE 36"h x 19"w x 14"d - FOR MSA EMERGENCY AIR MASK) - SIMILAR TO LABS SAFETY SUPPLY CO. AIR MASK MODEL 401 + WALL CASE A1441	
		2	CLOCK	

Fig. 7.1 Example of Room Data Sheet

60

DATE: 21 SEPT. 81
REV. 9 NOV 81
REV. 16 NOV 81
REV. 15 DEC 81
REV. 27 JAN 82

DATE APRVD :

APRVD BY :

MECHANICAL
- ☒ NORMAL COMFORT
- ☐ SPECIAL
  - TEMP —
  - HUMID —
  - OTHER —
- ☒ EQUAL
- ☐ NEGATIVE
- ☐ POSITIVE
- ☐ INDIVID RM CNTRL
- ☐ SPCL FILTER RQMTS
- ☒ ZONE TEMP CNTRL

LIGHTING
- ☒ COLOR CORRECT
- ☐ EMERGENCY
- ☒ FLUORESCENT
- ☐ ILLUMIN LVL —
- ☒ INCANDESCENT

POWER
- ☒ 110 v ac
- ☐ 220 v ac
- ☐ PHASE

1 FOR
15K WALL CASE

SWITCHES / OUTLETS
- ☐ CEILING
- ☒ CLOCK
- ☒ EMERGENCY
- ☐ EXPLOS PROOF
- ☐ FLOOR
- ☒ GROUNDED
- ☐ HANDING
- ☐ VAPOR TIGHT
- ☒ WALL
- ☐ WATER TIGHT
- ☐ X-RAY / PORTABLE

AMODATE
N HOLE TRAYS

COMMUNICATIONS
- ☒ COMPUTER TERM
- ☒ INTERCOM
- ☐ PAGING
- ☒ TELEPHONE
- ☐ TV - CLOSED
- ☐ TV - PUBLIC

PLUMBING
- ☒ ACID WASTE
- ☒ COUNTER SINK - DBL
- ☒ COUNTER SINK - SNGL
- ☐ CLINICAL SINK
- ☐ DSTLD H_2O
- ☒ EMERG EYE WASH
- ☐ EMERG SHWR
- ☐ FLOOR DRAIN
- ☐ LAVATORY
- ☐ SERV SINK - AUTO
- ☐ SERV SINK - FOOT
- ☐ SERV SINK - KNEE
- ☐ SERV SINK - JANITOR
- ☐ SERV SINK - PLASTER
- ☐ STEAM
- ☐ URINAL
- ☐ WATER CLOSET
- ☐ WATER CLOSET - HANDICAP

IFT LOCATION MAY
NORK COUNTER- ELEY 5.
2CHITECTURAL DW06.
2QUIPMENT PLAN/ELENS.
7ED TO PROVIDE 3-
VORK AREAS.

GASES
- ☐ NAT'L GAS
- ☐ COMP AIR
- ☐ VACUUM
- ☐ OXYGEN
- ☐ NITROGEN
- ☐ NITROUS OXIDE

FLOOR
- ☐ CARPET
- ☐ CONC
- ☐ RAISED
- ☒ RESILIENT TILE
- ☐ TERRAZZO
- ☐ VINYL
- ☐ WOOD

BASE
- ☐ CERAMIC TILE
- ☐ EPOXY
- ☒ RUBBER
- ☐ TERRAZZO

WALL
- ☐ CMU / EPOXY
- ☒ CMU / PAINT
- ☐ DRYWALL / EPOXY
- ☐ PAINT
- ☐ PLASTER
- ☐ VINYL
- ☐ W P PLASTER
- ☒ EXPOSED BRICK / EPOXY

CEILING
- ☐ AT / APPLIED
- ☒ AT / SUSPENDED
- ☐ EXPOSED STRUCT
- ☐ PLASTER

CEILING HT
- ☐ EXIST
- ☒ MIN   8°

DOOR SIZE
- ☒ HT   7°
- ☒ WIDTH   VARIES

FIRE ALARM
- ☐ CO 2
- ☐ DETECTOR
- ☒ PORT EXTING
- ☐ SPRINKLER
- ☒ EMERGENCY AIR MASK

SPCL CONDITIONS

MISCELLANEOUS

PERSONNEL
- ☒ AVG   14-16
- ☒ MAX   18-20
- ☒ FEMALE   90
- ☒ MALE   10

ROOM SIZE
- ☒ NSF   661
- ☐ GSF

SPACE SCHEMATIC PHASE

CONTROL DATA SHEET

PRESBYTERIAN HOSPITAL

PATHOLOGY / CLINICAL LABORATORIES

LEONARD MAYER   PLANNING CONSULTANT   RESTON, VA

PLAN 15

cause their primary purpose is to study combinations and alternatives in arranging all the components to achieve as ideal a configuration as possible.

These relationship diagrams can be done in varying levels of detail. For instance, one drawing may show the laboratory section as one block in relation to other sections in a hospital. Other sections to which the laboratory has a close relationship (i.e., surgery suite, outpatient entrance, and the morgue) will be shown directly adjacent to, or in proximity to the laboratory block. Sections with no relationship to the laboratory, such as social services or the gift shop, may be shown remotely. Strong positive and negative affinities are easily represented graphically with these types of drawings.

Relationship drawings (bubble diagrams) can and should be prepared for several levels of detail, by section, within each section, and perhaps even within each component of the laboratory. Their purpose is to communicate the essential relationships to complement the raw data developed in the space allocation program. Relationship drawings can be prepared easily by any member of the team with a good understanding of the interrelationships that the drawings should communicate.

Before proceeding to a schematic design, a thorough review and approval of all documents developed must be made. The scope of the project is now clearly defined and preliminary cost estimates can be developed by the architect or a contractor. The purpose of the review is to approve these documents and authorize the project team to proceed into schematic design.

This is an important review contractually. The architect must have assurance that the effort spent in proceeding into schematic design and further will not be wasted because the documents previously developed were inaccurate, incomplete, or otherwise inadequate.

FUNCTION OF THE LABORATORY 8

THE FIRST CONSIDERATION IN DESIGNING ANY FACILITY is the determination of the function of that facility. The knowledge of the laboratory's mission and projected function is essential. The main functions can be summarized as follows: assistance in making a diagnosis, confirmation of a diagnosis, assessment of clinical progress, assistance with prognosis, and assistance with control of therapy.

The essence of laboratory medicine is the acquiring of results by analytical procedures performed on patient specimens, the determination of the validity of the results, and the communication of information to the physician for making a diagnosis and treating the patient. The physician, patient, and laboratory are interrelated in a simplified cycle. The physician examines the patient and orders laboratory tests. The laboratory phlebotomist, nurse, or physician collects a blood, urine, fluid, or tissue specimen from the patient, and the laboratory staff analyzes the sample. The results are communicated to the physician, and treatment of the patient is based on those results.

A modern medical laboratory ordinarily is directed by a pathologist. In small hospitals it may be directed by a member of the medical staff with a pathologist as a consultant. The pathologist, a full member of the medical staff, reports directly to the administrator or Board of Trustees, depending on his contractual arrangement with the hospital. The pathologist is assisted in his direction of the laboratory by a chief technologist or business manager. This individual supervises several section supervisors. The laboratory often is divided into sections according to functionally related tests. Each of these sections is run by a section supervisor. Several functions may be combined into a single physical space. Instrument size, work volume, and the number of employees determine the number of sections. For each section, certain tests commonly are performed in high volume (Table 8.1).

> *" . . . The essence of laboratory medicine is the acquiring of results by analytical procedures performed on patient specimens, the determination of the validity of the results, and the communication of information to the physician for making a diagnosis and treating the patient. "*

Table 8.1

Routine tests that are commonly performed in relatively high volume in a community hospital.

CHEMISTRY & TOXICOLOGY

Albumin	LDH
Amylase	Osmolality
Bilirubin	pH
Blood, occult	Phosphatase, acid
Calcium	Phosphatase, alkaline
Carbon dioxide	Phosphorus
Chloride	Potassium
CPK	Protein, total
Creatinine	Sodium
Digoxin	Theophylline
Drug screen	Thyroxine
Gasses, blood	SGOT
Globulin	Triglycerides
Glucose	Urea nitrogen, (BUN)
Iron	Uric acid

HEMATOLOGY AND COAGULATION

Bleeding time	LE preparation
Blood count	Morphology of cells
Bone marrow	Platelet count
Clotting factors	Prothrombin time
Fibrin split products	Sedimentation rate
Fibrinogen	Thrombin time
Hemoglobin	Thromboplastin time
Hematocrit	

BLOOD BANK AND IMMUNOLOGY

Agglutinins, febrile	Blood typing
Antibody, qualitative	Coombs test
Antibody, quantitative	Globulin, Rh immune
Antinuclear antibodies	Platelet concentrate
Antistreptolysin O	Pregnancy test
Blood crossmatch	Syphilis serology

MICROBIOLOGY

Culture, bacterial	Ova and parasites
Culture, fungal	Sensitivity studies
Culture, tubercle	Smears

ANATOMIC PATHOLOGY AND CYTOLOGY

Autopsy	Frozen section
Cytopathology, fluid	Special stains
Cytopathology, smears	Surgical pathology
Consultation	

CLINICAL PATHOLOGY SECTIONS

Hematology Section

The primary activity of the hematology section usually is the study of cellular elements of the blood and, in most sections, blood coagulation. Tests performed in this section include the enumeration of different types of blood cells, structure and functional activity of blood cells, status and proliferative behavior of precursor cells in the bone marrow, and the role of blood vessels, platelet function, and blood coagulation in maintaining hemostatic integrity. The precise responsibilities of any given hematology section may vary greatly and should be defined for each laboratory as completely as possible before designing the section.

In an average general hospital, the hematology section can be expected to perform about 50 percent of the total number of procedures (raw count) conducted in that laboratory. However, this does not equate directly to space. Examination of the peripheral blood is performed on almost all patients because of the well-recognized importance of determining the presence of anemia, leukocytosis, and a variety of other abnormalities. This is relevant when considering traffic flow patterns and location of the hematology section in relation to other laboratory sections. Generally, the hematology section requires both counter space and sit-down counter heights because a considerable amount of the work performed in the section is done while seated.

A hematology section will not require unusual items in construction; however, it will require all the customary facilities, which include electricity, plumbing facilities, light, heating, air-conditioning, and ventilation. Adequate room should be provided for automated equipment as increasing demands have necessitated the development of sophisticated automated equipment that can handle accurately large volumes of work relating to enumeration of blood cell differentiation and coagulation. In some settings specimen procurement or phlebotomy is an activity of the hematology section.

Microbiology Section

The microbiology section performs those tests and procedures that isolate and identify the microorganisms causing infectious disease. Infectious organisms may be bacteria (bacteriology), fungi (mycology), parasites (parasitology), acid fast organisms (mycobacteriology), and viruses (virology). Not all laboratories provide the same level or number of microbiologic services. In this section, fluorescent microscopy and immunology or serology (detection of antigens or antibodies) also may be performed within this functional area. The variety and extent of services provided by the microbiology section depend on multiple factors including the size of the patient facility served, expertise and interest of personnel, availability of reference laboratories, and cost-effectiveness of test procedures. As with other functional areas of the laboratory, the degree of sophistication of test performance of the section must be established along with the extent and volume of test procedures to be performed. This will in turn impact on section size and design. In locating the microbiology functions within the laboratory area, local statutes relative to safety codes for adequate external venting must be met. The only laboratory area requiring close proximity would be glassware washing and sterilization areas, unless the microbiology section is large enough to incorporate these functions in its own area.

The hazards of contamination as well as employee safety are important factors in both the internal design of the microbiology suite and in its relationship with the remainder of the laboratory. It is generally accepted that the section should be some distance from the main entrance of the laboratory to limit the amount of traffic. An enclosed room provides more safety than an open one and it may be suggested that within that area, another enclosed room be available for handling more infectious materials, such as fungi and tuberculosis. The area should be equipped with laminar flow hoods and ultraviolet lighting to maintain sterility when not in use. In design, the section will require all the customary facilities of electricity, plumbing, lighting, and gas systems. Special needs include negative pressure air-conditioning and ventilation, and venting hoods that meet local statutory requirements. There needs to be an adequate communication system (sight, phone, intercom, or telewriter) between the section and other areas of the laboratory.

In designing a laboratory for microbiology the following areas may be considered separately:

- *Handling of specimens to include culturing and subculturing*
- *Isolation*
- *Staining and microscopic examination*
- *Media preparation*
- *Fluorescent microscopy*
- *Instrumentation*
- *Disposal*

Handling of Specimens

All specimens for culture are submitted to this area, where they are initially placed into culture media and identified. This work is performed most satisfactorily at sit-down benches where tedious work can be performed in more comfort. These benches should contain drawers for storage; storage space is dependent upon the volume of workload. For convenience, refrigeration and incubation facilities should be close at hand. For larger laboratories, these may be walk-in; for smaller laboratories, commercial type, nonfreezing units are desirable. Gas outlets are necessary for each technician area, and space must be available for tanks of gas for the CO_2 incubator. If culture media are prepared by the section, the preparation area should be near the specimen handling area.

Isolation

If possible, this area should be completely enclosed and away from the routine work flow of the section, but within the confines of the section perimeter. It should be as independent of other areas as possible so that infectious materials can be brought and confined there. Necessary equipment includes a hood, preferably a laminar flow variety, with proper ventilation and filtration. If this area is used only during certain periods of the day, a stand-up counter may be convenient. Gas, water, electrical outlets, and vacuum should be available. An ultraviolet light source may be useful to maintain a sterile area.

Staining and Microscopic Examination

Sit-down areas for microscopic work must be provided. These should be ample enough to provide room for microscopes and lamps, slides, writing materials, racks, and other accessories. The benches should be open underneath for leg room and it is convenient to have pullout drawers or overhead shelves for storage. This area should not be compromised because a considerable amount of employee time is spent here. Gas and electrical outlets are necessary. A staining sink equipped with special nozzle for washing slides as well as vacuum supply may be necessary. The size and placement of the sink will be an individualized preference.

Media Preparation

In approaching this important area, one must consider several points:

- *Storage of materials*
- *Preparation of media*
- *Sterilization*
- *Dispatch or storage of media*
- *Quality control*

This area should be as free from traffic flow as possible, yet be near areas of media dissemination, sterilization, and glass washing. Ample counter space must be provided, preferably of stand-up height, not only for preparation, but for overnight incubation and storage before refrigeration. An area may be necessary for packaging the final product for refrigerator storage or shipment to other destinations. Wall shelving plus cupboard and drawer space is necessary for storage of media and related supplies. No leg room is needed under the counters so they can be used to fullest capacity for storage. Autoclaves and hot-air sterilization must be nearby. At least one sink, preferably a double one, must be available along with gas and electrical outlets. It is convenient if this area is equipped with piped-in distilled water, and there may have to be arrangements for a special waterline for water demineralization if the distilled water is not of sufficient purity. Refrigeration and carts for carrying media must be available and space is required for these.

Fluorescent Microscopy

The main requirement of this area is that it be enclosed and completely free of light. For microscopic work, there must be a low bench with leg room underneath. If all the preparations for fluorescent microscopy are performed in this area, there should also be stand-up benches, a sink, storage areas, refrigeration, and incubation facilities. Electrical outlets are necessary.

Instrumentation

New instruments have been developed for microbiology, so in the design of a laboratory, consideration should be given to space for future equipment. Some of these instruments include the following:

1. *Bacterial detection devices using radioisotopes.*

2. *Turbidity-measuring equipment for dilution and standardization.*

3. *Automatic colony counting equipment.*

4. *Antibiotic sensitivity testing and, depending on the instrument, desired floor or bench space is necessary. There must be an access to water and electrical outlets.*

5. *Gas chromatography—bench space is necessary with ample room for a tank of helium gas and storage for accessories.*

Miscellaneous

Areas must be provided in microbiology for performance of tests such as parasitology preparation, antibiotic sensitivity testing, secretarial work, etc. Space allotted and bench structure will be dictated by work performed.

Disposal

All contaminated items must be disposed of in a manner that precludes dissemination of microbes. A small, easily disinfected area, or room, should be available with pans for autoclaving contaminated tubes. Also needed are garbage cans with sterilizable bags for disposal of petri dishes and other disposable contaminated materials. These should be autoclaved or incinerated. This area should be as isolated as possible from the routine work flow of the section.

Virology Section

Virology is the study of obligate, intracellular organisms unable to reproduce outside a living cell host. Viruses as a group are the single most common cause of human disease. The specific approaches to viral diagnosis include serologic studies (determination of antibodies), cytologic studies, demonstration of viral antigen by immunologic methods, isolation of viruses from tissue or body fluids in appropriate tissue culture, and direct examination by electron microscopy. Traditional diagnostic virology usually has been left to public health laboratories. Because of new methodology and techniques, it is now reasonable to consider diagnostic virology for direct patient management in the community-based hospital. This allows rapid etiologic diagnosis of viral infection with the possibility of specific therapy in mind.

The scope of services in this section depends on several important factors, such as size of the hospital, availability of funds, technical expertise of personnel, research facilities, and relevance of results from testing procedures. An area to be used for viral isolation must protect workers from infection as well as protect culture specimens from contamination. It should be in an area free of traffic and completely enclosed. The room should be well ventilated, air-conditioned, and have negative pressure to make certain that infectious particles do not escape into the environment. A well-exhausted and filtered biologic safety cabinet is mandatory for this room, particularly when processing tissues. Hoods with excellent filtration must be provided to prevent dissemination of viruses.

Ultraviolet light sources must be available for sterilization. Aerosols produced from the use of live antigens in inoculating culture media must be guarded against by using adequate disinfectants in isolated areas. Counter heights should accommodate sit-down microscopic work as well as stand-up work. These heights may depend on the personal preference of the employee.

Immunology Section

Immunology encompasses the detection of antigens or antibodies in various body fluids. It may be a separate section or overlap with blood bank, hematology, chemistry, immunoassay or serology activities. The design and size of this laboratory depends on the testing to be carried out and the volume of testing. It also depends on whether the immunology laboratory is completely independent or whether it is integrated into other sections with sharing of equipment. In general, activities in this section could include immunodiffusion, immunoelectrophoresis, fluorescent microscopy, automated equipment to measure various proteins, serologic techniques, and radioisotope work.

Nuclear Medicine Section

The nuclear medicine section is concerned with the diagnostic use of radioisotopes. The section encompasses two major areas: in vivo and in vitro studies. In vivo studies require injection of a radionuclide into a patient and subsequent nuclear scanning. In vitro studies are concerned with the diagnostic use of radionuclides to analyze blood samples for concentrations of various analytes. These two areas may be incorporated into one section or may be in separate sections. This depends on the qualifications of the director and his staff, and whether the responsibility of the nuclear medicine section falls under the supervision of pathology, radiology, internal medicine or various combinations of these three entities.

Generally, the nuclear medicine section should be in a separate area from the rest of the laboratory. The in vivo isotope area includes equipment to measure radioactivity that has been injected into a patient. Types of equipment may include a rectilinear scanner, scintillation gamma camera, and single probe with collimator. A computer may be incorporated for statistical and dynamic studies. Special considerations include electrical power with dedicated lines for each instrument, proper shielding and adequate water supplies for flushing radioactive materials, storage areas that can be used for disposal of isotopes, and adequate air exhaust or vacuum system for venting of radioactive gas studies into the atmosphere.

In some laboratories the in vitro area may be part of the chemistry section. In the in vitro area, little or no shielding is required since the exposure doses and materials used are insignificant even when stored in quantities sufficient for several weeks of work. Special considerations include an adequate supply of water for disposing of radioactive materials, areas for storing of radioactive materials for decay, and adequate electrical lines for radioactive counters.

Urinalysis Section

Urinalysis is the analysis of urine. It commonly encompasses the enumeration and identification of formed elements in the urine and the qualitative determination of common analytes. Routine urinalysis is one of the most commonly performed laboratory procedures; consequently, the section should be in a central location and conveniently located in relation to other high volume laboratory sections such as hematology and chemistry. The functions in the urinalysis section can be separated as follows:

- *Receipt and collection of specimen*
- *Specimen preparation*
- *Specimen examination*
- *Disposal of specimen*

Receipt and/or Collection of Specimens

Urine specimens often are collected elsewhere and brought to the laboratory. Since the specimens may not be examined immediately, it is necessary to store them to prevent deterioration. In order to do this, storage must be under refrigeration, and consequently, adequate refrigerator space must be provided for the number of specimens anticipated.

In most facilities some patients come directly to the laboratory where the specimen is collected. Therefore, toilet facilities are necessary and should be located as near as possible to the urinalysis section. Many laboratories provide a pass-through window from the toilet facility directly into the laboratory. This provides for minimum delay and maximum convenience.

As a part of the collection requirements, containers must be provided and storage space is necessary. In a large active laboratory, considerable numbers of these containers may be stored.

Specimen Preparation

Before beginning the actual analysis, specimens generally are arranged on a counter top where they may be numbered and correlated with report forms. A counter area must be provided for this purpose and of sufficient size to meet the requirements of the individual laboratory with ample space left over for unusually heavy workloads.

Specimen Examination

For the most part, examination may be conducted in the same area as the specimen preparation. A centrifuge is required as well as a separate area for microscopic examination. The counter for microscopic examination should be of desk height so that the work may be performed while seated. Some urine specimens require special examination and a separate laboratory bench area should be available for this. This area should be provided with basic facilities such as running water, electrical outlets, and gas. Ordinarily, the instruments that are required do not occupy a great deal of space; however, if unusual procedures are to be performed, the requirements for these must be recognized in advance and space provided.

Automated routine urinalysis equipment is now available and if its use is anticipated, proper bench space for this instrumentation should be incorporated into the laboratory design.

Specimen Disposal

The urine itself may, of course, be disposed of by flushing down the sink, and the used containers tend to accumulate in considerable numbers. If these are disposable, waste containers must be provided for disposal and space must be incorporated in the laboratory design for these containers. The containers should be positioned both for the convenience of the technician and for convenient removal from the laboratory.

If nondisposable containers are to be used, provision must be made for their transport to the washing area. This probably is most conveniently done by using a cart, and the design of the laboratory should provide space for such a transport facility.

Blood Bank Section

The function of the blood bank section is to collect, process, preserve, prepare, and distribute blood and blood components and to provide safe transfusion of blood products to patients. Each of these operations has become highly specialized and regulated, and requires well-trained personnel and expensive equipment. Providing all the services may not be practical for some laboratories and some of the services can be provided by regional blood centers. The type of work in this section depends on many factors including the type of patient mix, physician demands, finances, size of hospital, expertise of laboratory personnel, and availability of regional blood centers.

The hospital may have donor facilities. If the hospital obtains its own blood, the size of the donor facility will be related to the volume of blood collected. Some space in the donor facility has to be allocated to the administration and secretarial activity required to carry out donor recruitment. The donor facilities, if possible, should be near the blood bank proper. The blood bank requires easy access to and from the operating, emergency, and delivery rooms. The area should be easily accessible, yet secluded enough to preclude unnecessary and annoying intrusions. The processing of blood requires bench space for technician's work and space for floor centrifuges and refrigerators. Adequate electricity and plumbing are required. The section may separate a unit of whole blood into many components (red blood cells, platelets, cryoprecipitate, plasma, white blood cells, and coagulation concentrates). This processing requires adequate space and centrifugation. The section also may be involved in plasmapheresis. This process requires a large amount of space and can be done in the donor area.

Donor records, inventory control, patient records, records of blood release, transfusion records, and quality control records all require appropriate desk and file space. Administrative and clerical functions require desks, files, chairs, and casework for books and records.

Refrigerators are required for blood storage and preferably should have pullout or rotating shelves for easy access. Deep freezes and possibly liquid nitrogen is needed for frozen plasma and blood components. Appropriate space also must be provided for storage of blood fractions at room temperature. Rotators or some other method of providing agitation is needed for platelets. Proper alarms should be installed so that if the temperature of the storage units falls outside the appropriate range, prompt action can be taken. In the case of hospitals, this usually means that the alarm should ring at the switchboard or in a portion of the laboratory that is staffed with a 24-hour, on-site person.

Blood processing requires microscopes, centrifuges, refrigerators, illuminated boxes, heating blocks, water baths, cell washers, plasma expellers and, if frozen blood is handled, glycerolizing-deglycerolizing equipment. Work benches should be at sitting height and accompanied by appropriate casework providing cupboards, drawers, and shelves.

Chemistry Section

The primary function of the clinical chemistry section is to perform qualitative and quantitative analyses of body fluids such as blood, urine, and spinal fluid, as well as feces, calculi, and other materials. The common unit operations of clinical chemistry may include the following steps: obtaining the specimen, centrifugation, obtaining a measured sample, dilution, reagent addition, mixing, transferring, separation of desired constituent, reaction to form the compound to be measured, incubation, measurement of some property of the desired compound, calibration, quantification, and presentation of results. Any given procedure may not involve all of these steps or adhere to this order. These steps may be done manually or with automated instruments.

Chemistry procedures also can be divided into three separate areas: STAT, Routine, and Special. STAT tests must be done quickly and on demand. Routine tests are those most commonly done and results are needed in 24 hours or less. Special tests are complex tests that may be done in batch, one or more times per week in the laboratory, or may be sent to outside testing laboratories. The number of tests sent out obviously will influence the structure and design of the chemistry section.

The actual size of this section varies greatly depending on the size of the institution, and more importantly, on the patient mix. Also, it will depend on whether routine admission batteries are required, the number of hours the laboratory provides services, and the number of procedures offered. It may be desirable to set aside areas for a STAT or emergency laboratory, special studies, research and development, microchemistry for pediatric and geriatric patients, pulmonary function, reagent preparation, and special storage for the specialized glassware and supplies often required.

The decision regarding a central specimen collection and receipt area may require setting up this space in the chemistry section. The provision for these areas must take into account, perhaps more than in any other functional area, the economic and practical feasibility of performing everything in the laboratory, based primarily on the availability of qualified technical personnel and the presence of qualified professional supervision.

Obviously, the physical size of the section varies greatly. The usual error is overcrowding people. Planning should include an area for clerical functions where all current records, log books, and quality control charts are kept. Office areas may be included for the section supervisor.

All chemistry related functions should be kept within a contiguous area. Facilities should be kept as flexible as possible to allow easy introduction of new equipment and procedures. Usual requirements of heat, light, air, ventilation, air-conditioning, and possibly vacuum are necessary. Natural gas is unnecessary because open flames no longer are used. Purified bottled gases now are used and safe storage must be provided for them. Safety equipment, i.e., fire extinguisher, fire blankets, sprinkler systems, hoods, eye wash stations, etc., must be provided.

High purity deionized and/or distilled water must be provided. Refrigeration at 4°C to 8°C and freezer space of −20°C must be installed. A walk-in unit is sometimes necessary.

A separate automated laboratory section often is established in a hospital to run tests of sufficiently high volume or complexity, or perform tests that must be done as rapidly as possible in small or large volume groupings. A discussion of whether to automate a test is not within the scope of this chapter, but the question is one which realistically must be answered before an automated laboratory is set up. Automation in terms of large capital outlays for multitest capabilities may not necessarily be advisable. A distinct need should be shown and justification made on a realistic basis. The availability of automation at a regional facility may provide a better means of obtaining these procedures at substantial savings.

The size of the hospital, anticipated workload, availability of trained personnel, type of automation, degree of automation, manner of work flow, whether the laboratory is computerized, cost of equipment reagent preparation, and local service are all factors that play a part in the design and size of an automated laboratory.

Basically, the facilities should be located within the same functional area as all other chemistry tests. It should be of adequate size to accommodate the various pieces of equipment without crowding, especially to allow ready access to the equipment for servicing from all sides. The usual utilities, i.e., light, air-conditioning, heat ventilation, electricity, etc., must be provided. In addition, depending on the equipment, special electrical requirements may be necessary. Separate sewage and/or waste disposal as well as fume hoods, compressed gases, and air and distilled or deionized water connections may be advisable.

Adequate reagent storage and/or preparation areas should be provided. Adequate refrigerator/freezer space must be available as well as storage space for a supply of spare parts. In addition, adequate record handling and record storage space must be provided. A room set aside specifically for repair and maintenance of equipment and perhaps space for a full-time electronics and maintenance person may be necessary. Office spaces for a senior technologist and clinical chemist should be placed adjacent to this functional area.

STAT Laboratory

A STAT laboratory is a functional service concept designed to provide results within a required period of time, varying from a few minutes to a few hours. A STAT laboratory may be a separate physical space. In identifying the objectives of a STAT laboratory, some of the considerations are professional (pertaining to requirements for patient care), and others are operational (depending on special needs within the laboratory).

Operational considerations largely determine the configuration of a STAT laboratory. Most hospital laboratories mix STAT and routine tests. Commonly, a STAT laboratory is maintained at night and on weekends, using the same equipment for routine workload during the week. There are certain advantages to having a completely separate STAT laboratory, whether tests are ordered during routine working hours or at other times. In large, active general hospitals, STATs are significantly disruptive to smooth laboratory work flow, whether it be specimen collection, processing, performance of procedures, or reporting results. Therefore, it may be desirable to establish a separate STAT laboratory, to improve work flow patterns in both the routine and STAT areas, and to improve the effectiveness of both. This requires some duplication of equipment and facilities, although unnecessary duplication is largely avoided by having one area backup the other. To determine the professional considerations for the design of a STAT laboratory, it is necessary to know the kinds of patients

" . . . A STAT laboratory is a functional service concept designed to provide results within a required period of time, varying from a few minutes to a few hours. "

that are being treated and the particular requirements of the physicians responsible for their treatment. These considerations can make an enormous difference. For example, the laboratory for a large, general hospital which has an active emergency room has a great need for STAT procedures, particularly in the blood bank, hematology, and clinical chemistry sections.

Additionally, if the hospital has a hematology service concerned with the treatment of patients who have leukemia and other blood disorders, some special needs are generated. One of the most difficult problems is providing platelets for patients who need them. It is difficult to identify exact criteria for platelet transfusion and obtain platelet concentrates when necessary.

Another important factor is the kind of physicians in the hospital. Surgeons have different needs than internists. The number of pediatric patients is of great importance in deciding how much emphasis there should be on ultra-micro procedures. Also, the presence of a large house staff of relatively inexperienced physicians has great bearing on the number of STAT tests requested. These physicians tend to use the STAT test more frequently. If the hospital is active in treating shock patients, whether due to trauma, sepsis, or other causes, it must provide rapid coagulation studies to detect coagulation abnormalities. Obviously, a careful evaluation is essential to proper design of the STAT batteries, whatever they may be.

It is worthwhile to make some distinction between STAT requirements that occur primarily in hematology and chemistry and those that occur in blood bank. The blood bank can have an active service on a 24-hour basis, and STATs are nicely handled in the blood bank area without seriously disrupting other services. However, it may be necessary to have a separate STAT laboratory for hematology and chemistry, and this area should be combined in a single location. The general relationship to strive for is to locate the STAT hematology-chemistry laboratory immediately adjacent to both the routine chemistry and hematology laboratories. Except for those simple screening tests that can be performed in the STAT area, it is desirable to separate toxicology procedures that have special facility requirements.

Facilities Design

Although the STAT laboratory includes both chemistry and hematology, a division of samples and working areas is made after incoming specimens are identified and initially processed. Mostly, the type of specimen, i.e.,

Table 8.2

Other functional and support areas frequently found in medical laboratories.

TEACHING AND RESEARCH PROGRAMS

    Offices
    Conference rooms
    Research and training laboratories

ADMINISTRATIVE SUPPORT

    Offices
    Stenographic and secretarial offices
    Conference rooms

EMPLOYEE SUPPORT

    Offices in each department for supervisors
    Lounges
    Restroom facilities

INSTRUMENT REPAIR AND MAINTENANCE

PATIENT SUPPORT

    Waiting rooms
    Phlebotomy
    Patient examining and procedure rooms
    Restrooms

CENTRAL STORAGE AND SUPPLY

---

blood vs serum, is different and nothing is to be gained by complete integration. In fact, separation allows a smoother work-flow pattern provided the space and its arrangement are adequate. Obviously, such design depends on the kinds of tests to be done and the methods and equipment used to do them.

One should consider the arrangement of the laboratory and some important features about the movement of specimens through it. Generally, those higher volume tests that need to be done most rapidly should be located in an area immediately adjacent to the clerical processing part of the laboratory. Those tests that are done less frequently or require special equipment or furniture, such as the pediatric ultramicro procedures and the sit-down benches for microscopy, should be located further away.

Relatively few STATS are required in life-threatening situations. These include blood and urine glucose, serum potassium, packed cell volume, examination of blood smears, blood gases, typing and cross-matching blood, and some toxicology measurements. In addition, determination of clotting factors in patients who are suspected of having disseminated intravascular coagulation, and examination of cerebrospinal fluid, may be necessary on a STAT basis in order to prevent serious complications and possible death from underlying disorders. Frequently, use of other tests depends on the need and desire of a physician to have results so he can monitor the patient and begin treatment.

Instrumentation

Instrumentation is as variable as the kind of tests done. Almost no instruments are designed primarily or exclusively for STAT work, and those that are have limitations.

Larger laboratories may use automated equipment. Smaller laboratories probably will resort to manual methods. Advantages can be gained by using testing kits which are available for most STAT tests done, except for sodium, potassium, blood gases, and pH. Kits vary considerably according to manufacturer and even from lot to lot, so it is necessary to have a good evaluation of the accuracy that can be obtained with them. Even large laboratories will find kits a real advantage in some circumstances, particularly as a way of saving personnel time, which is always a major problem in a STAT laboratory.

ANATOMIC PATHOLOGY SECTIONS

Histology Section

The function of a histology section is to process tissue, removed surgically or at autopsy, for microscopic examination and diagnosis. It should be close to the pathologist's office. This is necessary for the fairly extensive communication which is required for routine tissues and also for rapid performance of frozen sections. The activities of the histology section generally begin when the various tissue specimens are received. This area should provide sufficient counter and desk space so that the necessary clerical functions can be performed. Generally, the gross examination also is conducted in this or an immediately adjacent area which requires further counter space, running water, adequate lighting, dictating equipment, and sufficient space for storage of tools, gowns, gloves, and containers of fixative solutions.

The area in which these activities are conducted must have excellent forced ventilation, because the most common fixative is formaldehyde. This will be present in considerable quantities in this room and if there is not adequate ventilation, the room will be uninhabitable. Additionally, some of the specimens may contain pathogenic organisms and it is desirable to have a suitable hood and facilities for performing cultures.

After the specimens have been examined grossly and sections taken for microscopic examination, it is necessary to store the gross specimens for varying periods of time. At the very least, sufficient space should be provided to permit storage for two weeks. Some laboratories that store specimens for a longer period of time require considerably more space. Again, since considerable quantities of formaldehyde are generally used, there must be an adequate ventilation system with a continuous flow of fresh air. The area also requires adequate shelving and lighting.

Once the tissue sections have been selected for microscopic examination, usually they are placed in an automatic tissue processor for which space and exhaust ventilation must be provided. Of course, the number of processors depends on the number of specimens to be processed, and information concerning this can be obtained from the pathologist.

On completion of the automatic processing, the tissues then go to an embedding area and later to the microtome sectioning area. These activities are most conveniently conducted by technicians who are sitting; consequently, the counter height should be adjusted accordingly.

After the cutting process, the slides are dried and stained. Staining may be manual or automatic; however, in either case, space and exhaust ventilation must be provided for the necessary equipment. After staining, the slides are cover-slipped and labeled, which requires a sitting height bench top area, the size of which depends on the number of slides. This area should be well illuminated.

After the slides have been examined, it is necessary to have sufficient space to store the slides and also to store the paraffin blocks. In the case of slides, one of the main problems is the relatively great weight which develops when large numbers of slides are stored. For this reason, reinforced flooring is desirable. Paraffin blocks must be stored at a controlled temperature to prevent deterioration.

There are additional special requirements which are encountered in a histology section. Space must be provided for the performance of frozen sections. This is usually not a large space and needs no special comment, except that when the laboratory and surgical areas are separated from one another, it is convenient to establish a frozen section laboratory in the surgery suite. When this is done, a number of facilities must be duplicated to examine gross specimens, to stain specimens, and also to perform a microscopic examination at the site at which the frozen section is performed.

Another requirement in a histology section is for special stains and other special processing, such as decalcification. Areas should be provided for these activities that are separate from those provided for the routine work. Special reagents and glassware are needed and, in some instances, special equipment is required.

Still other special features may be needed from time to time in certain laboratories such as the ability to prepare celloidin specimens, specimens for electron microscopy, and other special procedures. Since these become specialized, detailed information regarding them need to be obtained from the pathologist or equipment planner.

Autopsy Section

Since the morgue and autopsy room are an integral part of the anatomic pathology section, and this section also relies on the resources of hematology, chemistry, microbiology, and clinical microscopy, the morgue and the autopsy room should be a part of the hospital clinical laboratory.

Morgue (body storage facility)

The morgue should be located with direct access from the elevator-corridor network and easy access to the exit used for body removal from the institution. The general arrangement should permit these functions to be accomplished with some privacy.

The requirements needed for body storage can be established by the inpatient load and the mortality rate in the hospital. Refrigeration is the accepted system for temporarily preserving a body. Refrigeration can be accomplished by either using enclosed refrigerated units which contain sliding, rolling carriers to move a mortuary tray into or out of the refrigerated unit or a specially constructed refrigerated room known as a cold crypt into which litter carts can be moved.

81

Autopsy Room

At autopsy the organs are removed from the body and dissected. Suitable specimens for morphologic, chemical, or microbiological examinations are removed. Photography is used commonly as a means of recording the gross findings and for teaching purposes.

The autopsy room would contain the autopsy table or tables, sinks, cabinets for storage of instruments, records, and specimens and accessory facilities such as scales for weighing tissues and bodies, recorder for dictation, x-ray viewing box, photography, and a small blackboard. The allocated space should allow at least 5 ft of area on each side of the autopsy table. There should be sufficient room for physicians, students, or nurses to observe the autopsy and inspect the organs. In larger teaching institutions a moveable stand for this purpose may be appropriate.

The room should be constructed so that sanitary cleanliness can be maintained. An adequate plumbing system should be installed with an excellent drainage system. The room should have adequate ventilation and be air-conditioned for temperature control. Lighting should be diffused with an accessory overhead reflector lamp for closer body examination.

There should be a small room adjoining the autopsy room where the pathologist may dress for the autopsy. This facility should include a shower and a storage area for disposable caps, gowns, and aprons and a waste container for their disposal.

Cytology Section

Cytology is the processing and study of exfoliated cells to determine morphologic abnormalities. It usually is incorporated into the section of histology for sharing facilities such as preparation of cell blocks. Cytology may be a separate section in some institutions and it is preferable to have it in close proximity to the histology section. Specimens received consist of smears already prepared, as well as various body fluids from which preparations are to be made. Special needs in this section include adequate ventilation with hoods to vent toxic fumes and adequate counter space with plumbing for sinks. In some circumstances vaginal, cervical, or other smears may be collected in the section and a suitable patient examining room for this purpose will be needed. If the cytology section is part of the general clinical laboratory, the examining room of the outpatient facility may be used.

Electron Microscopy Section

The electron microscope is a powerful instrument used to study the ultrastructure of various cells in a tissue from which conclusions are made regarding a disease process. Not every laboratory will have or need electron microscopy capability. In general, the area set aside for the installation of an electron microscope must be free from building vibrations and must have at least 10-ft ceilings. The environment for the electron microscope requires adequate electricity, plumbing, and air-conditioning. Adjacent space should be set aside for tissue preparation and photographic film processing. Procedures performed in an electron microscopy section fall into two categories: (1) Tissue Processing and Preparation, and (2) Microscopy and Photography Processing.

COMPUTERIZATION AND TELECOMMUNICATIONS

The laboratory, whether in a large urban medical complex or a small community hospital, most likely will become involved in automated data processing as a result of rapidly expanding computer and microcomputer technology. The specific functions that a laboratory computer system performs include printing lists of patient information for use in the laboratory, entering lists of tests requested for a patient, printing labels and specimen collections lists, updating the laboratory specimen accession records, and printing laboratory documents that indicate what test procedure to run on patient specimens. Additional functions include entering laboratory results into the computer via clinical laboratory instruments or manually, storing laboratory results, printing and distributing laboratory reports, sending patient charges to the billing office, printing workload reports for laboratory personnel evaluations, collating various laboratory data for each patient in a logical manner, generating quality control data and statistics, maintaining inventory, and producing workload recording statistics.

" . . . The laboratory most likely will become involved in automated data processing."

The practical use of computer technology in the clinical laboratory is expanding at a phenomenal rate. A computer system has two essential components for complete operation. The hardware component is the physical structure of the computer which includes the central processing unit, peripheral memory storage, and input devices. The software component is a program of instructions for the computer. Adequate space is needed for the various input and output devices such as CRTs with keyboards, printing terminals, line printers, and mark sense readers.

Communications, both written and verbal, are a major component of all medical care. The essence of laboratory medicine is acquiring results by analytical procedures performed on patient specimens and the communication of the results to the physician for making a diagnosis and treating the patient. Telecommunications refer to the transmission of data over a distance. The laboratory may use noncomputer means of telecommunications or may develop a computer system with telecommunications capability. The net effect of telecommunication is a marked decrease in turnaround time from specimen collection to data dissemination.

Interface of the computer with laboratory instrumentation usually is of little consequence to room placement as this interface is achieved by the use of cabling. The vendor of the selected computer system should be asked if there are any constraints on cable lengths.

The most important interface affecting room placement is between the computer and the people who customarily use the system. The computer should be a well-understood, visible, and easily accessible tool. For example, if the system software provides for keyboard entry of manual test results or provides computational subroutines at the main computer console, then some means must be provided to allow personnel to enter the computer room and perform these functions. The availability of remote input and output terminals and the functional capability of the software makes room placement proportionately less critical.

Large volumes of printed reports from line printers, such as periodic ward reports, require space for clerical personnel to disassemble the continuous form report paper and remove carbon interleaves. Such activity should occur in a remote or adjacent area of the computer room that has a direct exit from the laboratory itself.

Ideally, laboratory personnel should be provided with easy access to the input side of the room. Outputs should be directed out the opposite side of the room into the hospital proper. The presence of remote input or output terminals reduces the volume of such traffic but will not invalidate this principle.

Environmental control and the cost of such control may be reduced by placing the computer room away from exterior walls of the building. If the computer is physically placed near an exterior wall containing large expanses of glass, more extensive air-conditioning capability is required, although short periods of temperature extremes may occur and cause intermittent computer malfunctions.

Space Requirements

The size of the computer room depends entirely on the type of equipment to be installed. Consult the prospective equipment vendor for assistance in this area. Evaluate decisions regarding adequate size by contacting other laboratories that have similar hardware and that are working towards similar organizational goals.

Presenting rules of thumb for square-foot requirements to house facilities or functions is, at best, a dangerous proposition and will not be attempted. However, those who are presently planning new laboratory facilities without concurrent computer installation, but anticipating such installation in a year or two, may find that from 225 sq ft to 275 sq ft of computer room space may be required for a typical present day turnkey system. Proceed at your own risk in determining possible space requirements for undefined future computer installations.

Room Construction

Normal office-type construction is acceptable. Employment of fire-resistant or noncombustible materials is not mandatory; however, their use is encouraged. Computer peripheral equipment, especially line printers and teletypes, contribute to high noise levels, and consequently, acoustical deadening material should be used wherever possible.

Determine in advance the overall dimensions and weights of the computer hardware to be installed, as special provision may be needed to move the equipment from the receiving dock to the computer room. Doors must be wide enough, as must bends and turns in halls and stairwells. Elevators should be checked for size and weight limitations. Check with the equipment vendor to determine how the components will be shipped and if there is any flexibility in packaging. These components usually are shipped on wooden pallets and are subject to a vendor requirement that they be unpacked by, or in the presence of, a vendor service representative. A nonstandard shipment package configuration may be requested to ease any transport problems within a specific institution.

Floors

Many turnkey computer systems presently available do not require the installation of raised floors to facilitate the routing of power supply cables, etc.

However, if future additions to equipment configurations are anticipated or a greater degree of component placement flexibility within the computer room is desired, it may be wise to consider the installation of a raised floor at the outset. Consult the equipment vendor to determine if a raised floor is required.

Raised floors may be constructed by a general contractor or purchased from companies specializing in computer installation fixtures. Construction can be of steel, aluminum, or fireproof wood. The free-access type is recommended over other types as it provides greater cable placement options. Regardless of source, there should be no exposed metal surfaces on the raised floor as this could constitute an electrical safety hazard and a potential source of static electricity. Ten pounds per square foot must be added to the conventional floor loading factor to compensate for the weight of the raised floor itself.

Regardless of what type of floor construction is used, the floor loading rates that computer equipment usually require must be considered. Most office-type construction floors are rated at 50 lb/sq ft for live load with an allowance of 25 lb/sq ft for partition loads. This may not be adequate for initial installation or may prove to be inadequate after future expansion of facilities. Consult the equipment vendor and architect on both new and remodeling construction plans.

Floor Surfaces

This section applies to conventional and raised floor construction. Floor covering material can contribute to the buildup of electrical static charges that cause discomfort for employees and may cause malfunction to electronic equipment. These static buildups can be minimized by using floor tile or other floor surfaces that have a maximum resistance of 2×10^{10} ohms, measured between the floor surface and the building. NFPA Standard No. 56, Chapter 25, Section 2522 has more detailed information.

Carpet floor coverings should be made of material that has the antistatic properties manufactured into the material rather than treated with antistatic agents after manufacture. These treatments may have a short effective life and may require retreatment frequently. Carpet users must pay for a more intensive maintenance program for controlling dust.

Lighting

A minimum average illumination of 40-foot candles measured at 30 in above the floor should be maintained in any area where printed material must be read by employees in the customary performance of their normal function. Direct sunlight should be avoided because of its extreme variability and the need for the low light levels necessary to observe various computer console lights, cathode ray tube images, etc. Lighting control should be sectionalized so that general levels of illumination can be controlled in areas of the room if desired.

Additional Space Requirements

The laboratory computer system operation may need additional computer-related space, the amount of which will vary depending on hardware installed, the contractual relationship concerning software responsibility with the equipment vendor, and the overall organizational goal of the laboratory.

Service Area or Room

An additional room, or an equivalent area in or near the computer room, is useful for vendor service personnel. This area is for storing test equipment, parts, electrical component schematics, etc. No size requirements can be stated for this service area; however, one vendor specified a minimum of 100 sq ft. Check with the equipment vendor for advice or assistance.

Programmer Rooms

Contractual responsibility for computer systems software varies from vendor to vendor. Some vendors assume full responsibility for currently operational software and promise the development and introduction of new applications packages at some future time. Other vendors provide the hardware only, and the laboratory must take full responsibility for software development. In the former case, it might be assumed that no programmer space would ever be required. In reality, some laboratories find that they have needs for computing applications that will not be satisfied by their software contract, or they develop interests that are outside the clinical laboratory applications being planned by their vendor, i.e., research interest, administrative applications, etc. It may be wise to consider allotting space for future programming efforts.

In the latter case, there will be a definite need for programmer office space, the extent of which is difficult to determine. Organizational goals, equipment configuration, availability of canned software components, and the implementation time schedule are all variables affecting space requirements for programming. A typical programmer office should be isolated from operational activity and noise. It should contain a reasonably large pedestal desk, a two-drawer file cabinet, 9 linear ft of bookshelf for 10-in × 12-in instructional materials, a chair, and should be about 100 sq ft in size. Programmer offices need not be close to computer rooms; however, this is desirable if possible.

Space for Storage of Supplies

Storage of report paper and magnetic media (disks and tape) ideally should be in areas that have environmental conditions identical to that of the computer room. It may be a separate room made for this purpose or the computer room may be used after installing appropriate metal storage fixtures. Additional precautions must be observed in storing magnetic tape. Reels should be stored in self-sealing, dust-proof cases, placed in the vertical position on racks providing partitions between reels, and remote from any source of magnetic flux greater than 50 oersteds.

Space for Storage of Computer Software and Laboratory Master Records

An often overlooked fact at many computer installations is that magnetic media containing systems software or master records represent investments of thousands of dollars in man hours required to develop them. A simple fire loss of an only copy of a systems program on a $4.50 magnetic disk could be an actual loss of $10,000 to $20,000. The same could be true if a large file of patient master records had to be reconstructed.

Prudence dictates an operational policy of maintaining duplicate backup sets of systems software and master records. These duplicates should be stored in protected storage areas as defined by NFPA Standard No. 75, Sections 300 and 600. Laboratory design should provide adequate amounts of such storage space. Off-premise storage sites may be considered if the required facility is or will not be available in the laboratory. At any rate, the value of the intelligence contained on those seemingly insignificant reels of tape should not be underestimated.

Fire and Safety Considerations

An overall program for fire prevention, fire control, and employee safety should be considered while planning the entire laboratory. The following suggestions are made concerning the computer area; however, other areas of the laboratory may also benefit from these suggestions. In any case, there must be compliance with the College of American Pathologists Inspection and Accreditation Commission on Fire Safety Standards, and other governmental building and fire codes.

If an overhead sprinkler system is used, a dry pipe system is recommended. This type of system, on detection of a fire, turns off all electrical power sources in the area before opening valves to fill the overhead sprinkler system. A battery-operated emergency light source should be provided to aid personnel in dealing with the situation.

If an automated carbon dioxide fire protection system is used, an alarm mechanism should be built into the system to warn personnel that the carbon dioxide has been released. Portable carbon dioxide cylinders may be used to supplement an automatic system or may be used as a primary extinguishing system if local regulations allow. A standpipe or hose unit should be located within effective range of the computer areas as a secondary extinguishing agent for a Class A Hazard. For additional information, refer to NFPA Standard No. 75.

If power connections are made beneath raised floors, waterproof receptacles and connectors should be used. The raised floor framing, if metal, also should be provided with an adequate earth ground to prevent shock hazards at all times. Emergency power controls for disconnecting the main power service to computer equipment should be convenient to the computer operator at his customary work station and also next to each exit door from the computer room.

Contact an insurance agent or underwriter and equipment vendors for assistance in fire and safety planning as the vendor can specify requirements and the insurance people can suggest approaches that will minimize risk and perhaps minimize insurance premiums. The insurance underwriter may also help to interpret applicable provisions of the Williams-Steiger Occupational Safety and Health Act of 1970 as they apply to the clinical laboratory setting.

Cabling Considerations for Automated Instruments and Computer Terminals

Cable to connect laboratory instrumentation and computer input/output

89

terminals to the computer is generally furnished by the equipment vendor. Installing and physically routing the cable usually is the responsibility of the purchasing institution. During the planning stage, work closely with the equipment vendor to determine cable sizes, length constraints, and any other requirements that may be necesessary.

Some general principles may be stated in planning for cable routing and installation. Cable lengths should be as short as possible to minimize electrical resistance and the potential electrical signal noise factor. Cabling must not run parallel to any high voltage or noise-producing devices such as fluorescent lamps or isolation transformers. If it is necessary to cross power lines with interface cables, the power lines should be crossed at right angles one foot on either side of the noise-producing device.

Do not plan to use tubular electrical conduit in the routing of cable. Although the cables usually are low-voltage, communication-type wires of a relatively small diameter, the cable connector plugs are of a much larger diameter. Removing and replacing these connectors to facilitate pulling the cable through the conduit is both difficult and unwise.

It is better to install a grid system of rectangular sheet metal duct work into the ceiling of all rooms in the laboratory that will initially or eventually house automated laboratory instrumentation or computer terminals requiring direct interface to the computer. This grid approach provides unlimited equipment placement flexibility. Placing this duct work grid in the floor should be avoided as laboratories have found that this is not nearly as flexible an arrangement. Placement of the master junction of this duct work grid in the computer room will depend on whether there is a raised floor in the computer room itself. If there is a raised floor, route the junction entrance into the room below floor level so as to further distribute the cables under the floor. If there is a conventional floor, use the same ceiling grid duct work arrangement in the computer room that was used in other areas of the laboratory.

Instrumentation cable grounds usually are isolated from the computer ground to avoid creating noise voltage differences. Using multiple grounds on a cable also can cause electrical noise and should be avoided. It is rarely possible to achieve complete suppression or isolation of noise. A grounding system should be installed that is itself isolated from electrical noise so as not to contribute to the problem. It should have a maximum of 3 ohms resistance to the connection to moist earth. See the Power Supply section of this chapter for earth grounding techniques.

Environmental Considerations

Consult the equipment vendor to obtain specific environmental requirements while in the planning stages as there are some variations between vendors in this area.

The ideal computer room has a regulated air-distribution system that provides cool, filtered, and humidity-controlled air. The room temperature is between 60°F and 80°F with a fluctuation of no more than perhaps 10°F in one hour. The relative humidity should be maintained between 40 percent and 60 percent, 78°F maximum wet bulb, with no condensation. System reliability decreases if these tolerances are exceeded over long periods of time. Probably the most important environmental factor affecting system performance is the rate and range of variability. A constant, consistent environmental state is the least troublesome although the high or low side of the specifications are approached or even exceeded.

Heat dissipation of all laboratory instrumentation, lighting fixtures, refrigerators, personnel, and computer equipment must be considered when determining the required air-conditioning capacity necessary for the laboratory. For example, the computer alone may dissipate as much as 20,000 BTUs per hour on some of the larger installations.

Creating positive air pressure in the computer room that is 0.1 in to 0.2 in of water above that of the surrounding area has been found useful in inhibiting dust and fume infiltration. This could be important in the laboratory. It has been found that heavy concentrations of sulfide fumes or chemicals that increase the presence of chloride ions in the air will impair the operation of and shorten the life of the computer. Chemicals or chemical combinations which in any way deteriorate Kyanar, Mylar, or irradiated PVC electrical insulation should be avoided. A high concentration of particulate matter in the air makes use of magnetic tape and disks, which are troublesome because their magnetic character naturally attracts electrically charged particles.

Power Supply Considerations

The nature of the power supply required to operate the computer can only be specified by its manufacturer. Some typical specifications for turnkey systems are the requirement of an independent power source of 117 V, single-phase, 60-cycle service of 2,000 W with a voltage fluctuation of no more than ±7 V.

Whatever the needs in this area, the most important consideration is the need for a source that is as free as possible from voltage fluctuations. Many items of electrically operated equipment in a hospital could easily, by themselves or starting in unison, cause severe voltage fluctuations of excessive duration (e.g., the simultaneous starting of a heating plant motor, an x-ray camera, and the morgue refrigerator). Power drops, only milliseconds in duration, can cause havoc during certain computer functions. Electrical storms also may be a source of interference to consistent power supply. It has been found in most laboratories that the usual auxiliary power supply in hospitals is of little use during total power failures because of the time required for the auxiliary to start.

Practical experience has shown that the greatest amount of difficulty arises when power fluctuation occurs during computer input or output transfers of information to auxiliary storage devices. The loss of all information contained on a disk storage unit can be catastrophic because both operating programs and all patient data may be lost.

Laboratories and equipment vendors have attempted to solve this problem by building safeguard features into the software operating systems whenever possible, by installing buffer motor generators, and by installing large capacitors. Answers to these problems must be sought in advance from equipment vendors, and the public utility supplying power.

Computer Hardware Grounding

Improper grounding of hardware configuration elements can influence performance significantly. The computer itself can be a noise source within the low-level signal collection input circuits used for online collection of data. The computer manufacturer probably has provided a sufficient grounding circuit for all hardware components within the power supply cord itself. An adequate insulated ground circuit must be available from the power supply panel to the nearest stable ground by the shortest most direct path possible.

Steel framing or the cold water piping system in the building may be used for a ground source. However, the continuity of metallic conduct must not be broken between the ground connection and earth, and electrical current flow must not be induced in beams or pipes from other electrical equipment within the hospital.

If these grounding methods are impossible or unacceptable, a grounding rod of .625 in or larger in diameter must be driven to a depth of 12 ft, or a metallic plate approximately 16 sq ft in surface area must be buried in moist earth.

MEDICAL LABORATORY DATA BASE 9

PRESENTLY, NO COMPLETELY SATISFACTORY AND USEFUL FOR-MULA EXISTS which relates total workload, hospital bed numbers, or patient days to the optimum gross or net square footage required by the laboratory. Good laboratory design depends on the presence of a complete functional plan that can only be developed from a useful clinical laboratory data base. This data base then is the framework on which all future decisions depend. It must include not only numbers concerned with test and unit workload, but also information indicating important aspects of laboratory service philosophy and any special circumstances that may exist within the institution.

A laboratory data base consists of all information available in a laboratory that might impact on the planning and design process. Examples of this include test volume, number of personnel, workload, number of beds, etc. Often, this information is readily available. In other instances, however, it takes considerable effort to gather. The development and maintenance of the clinical laboratory data base is an essential part of the planning process. To be useful, these data must provide meaningful information to all members of the planning team. Statistical information derived in a haphazard manner or without an understanding of its use represents an unproductive effort.

Data base groupings change as laboratory functional activities change, and those that were apparently satisfactory several years ago may not be meaningful when a current planning process begins. Additionally, headings or groupings useful in the planning of a general service laboratory will not necessarily be adequate when a specialized facility is contemplated.

The collection of the data base elements is not in itself a difficult activity but interpretation may become so if a careful review of the data early in the planning process is not instituted. In this way, it is possible to relate the data base to the functional plan so that there is a good understanding of why these data were collected and the manner in which these data impact on the functional plan itself.

" . . . No completely satisfactory and useful formula exists which relates total workload, hospital bed numbers, or patient days to the optimum gross or net square footage required by the laboratory."

It is important that the laboratory director determine the level of knowledge of the architect/planner and not presume the presence of an understanding that does not exist. The architect/planner must realize the tremendous change that has occurred with respect to methodology, instrumentation, and data processing, and that little useful reference material exists.

The architect/planner also has a responsibility to determine, early in the planning process, the level of understanding and interest with which the laboratory director approaches the new development. Assurance that the laboratory team is of the highest possible caliber is necessary. The laboratory director should provide knowledgeable and interested staff for the planning team, and the architect/planner will note involvement by laboratory staff members who have special duties in future test and workload planning. The architect/planner will be aware that each sectional area has been challenged to provide information regarding future instrumentation and the assistance has been sought and obtained from professional colleagues as a result of correspondence or site visitation. In this way, the laboratory directors have an opportunity to learn first-hand details of the successes and failures of their colleagues in the relationship of the data base to the functional plan of the completed facility.

The Data Base—General

1. Administrative
2. Clinical
3. Anatomic
4. Educational
5. Employee support
6. Laboratory support

The number and functions of administrative and other personnel requiring separate work spaces are an important part of the data base information. Adequate office area is necessary for managers, planners, and coordinators as well as for the director, other laboratory scientists, charge technologists, and senior technology personnel. Just as some staff do not require an enclosed work area, others must be provided with a soundproof environment.

The final plan depends on the inclusion within the data base of such information as the number of students in each year of training and the number of instructors. Educational philosophy determines the need for library space, pres-

> **"** . . . The collection of the data base elements is not in itself a difficult activity but interpretation may become so if a careful review of the data early in the planning process is not instituted. **"**

ent or absent, unique or shared, and the existence of separate student training areas in each section of the laboratory.

General hospital and/or laboratory policies determine whether a special lounge or coffee area is required and whether change rooms are located centrally or within each section. The total number of staff and local building codes makes possible the determination of adequate washrooms.

Laboratory policy also determines the design features of wash-up, sterilization, pure water supply, and storage facilities. Total staff numbers involved in these support activities and the volume of work to be done or the supply needed also play an important part.

It is important to emphasize that conceptual as well as numeric information should reside in the data base. Interpretation of numeric data alone leads to an incomplete functional plan.

The Data Base—Workload

The College of American Pathologists' Workload Recording Method provides a method which uses the following elements and can constitute a portion of a comprehensive data base.

1. Raw count (tests) – total, department, shift

2. Units – total, department, shift

3. Number of specimens collected

4. Number of STAT orders – total, department, shift

5. Number of routine orders – total, department, shift

6. Percentage of raw count – department, shift

Effective planning, just as effective management, requires an assessment of current levels of activity. Also necessary is a review of past experience and a projection of future trends. These data are best acquired through the application of the CAP Workload Recording Method which is an ongoing and dynamic activity.

In general, more planning information can be derived from test data than from unit data. It is important, however, to realize that the number of specimens to be collected influences the design of the accession area, and those locations used for tray and supply storage. Strategies outlining such matters as central or sectional accessioning require notation.

Knowledge of the total and shift STAT workload makes it possible to determine the size of the specialized STAT laboratory work area if this concept of service forms part of the laboratory philosophy. Should the plan be to perform STAT tests in the main work area, the numbers are perhaps less important.

The Workload Recording Method provides the laboratory director with a measure of personnel efficiency which encompasses variation in design, instrumentation, and overall laboratory policy and practice. It forms an essential part of the data base collection and can be used when forecasting future trends. Sometimes this is on the basis of past performance and at others depends on an expected change in functional activity or methodology. A variation in patient mix in the future can be studied with workload recording data. An increase in beds or a change in health care planning philosophy also can be assessed in this way.

The Data Base—Bed Size and Patient Days

While important in a general sense, the information derived from data concerning total bed capacity of an institution or the number of patient days per annum cannot be applied with great significance during the planning process. What is most important, of course, is the size and character of the laboratory workload.

The Data Base—Laboratory Features

1. Laboratory type

2. Patient type
   - *outpatient tests*
   - *inpatient tests*
   - *referred out tests*
   - *referred in tests*

3. Test type
   - *blood bank*
   - *clinical chemistry*
   - *hematology*
   - *histology*
   - *immunology*
   - *microbiology*
   - *nuclear medicine*
   - *urine and feces*
   - *special procedures*
   - *miscellaneous*

4. Instrumentation
   - *floor space*
   - *bench space*

In this important segment of the data base, numeric and conceptual data are required again in order to develop a satisfactory functional plan.

Data concerning the outpatient patient collection and test load properly interpreted allow for the provision of a patient reception and collection site of

98

adequate size. Should the test list include those requiring long waits or special nursing care, such as glucose tolerance or hormone analyses, additional features are included in the functional plan.

In addition to consideration of size, the location of the outpatient facility will be influenced by the need to share with another section of the hospital and such features as ease of street access to parking.

A heavy referral load requires special mail or courier facilities which would not be found in a laboratory not providing this type of service, yet perhaps performing the same number of total tests. If many specimens are to be referred out, attention will be drawn to the need for a special preparation area.

Designation of the test types in each section of the laboratory along with an understanding of the equipment configuration expected is a most useful exercise. It is in this area of planning that the greatest changes have occurred. Raw test counts give little information alone in this context. The planner must know the number, service, and physical features of each expected new automated instrument of significant size. If the data are accurate, the planner can determine the optimum location of this equipment within each section of the laboratory by using a functional flow diagram.

The Data Base—Data Processing and Telecommunications

Modern planning requires that special attention be given to the question of data processing and telecommunications. Consideration of this situation cannot be done in isolation, as a continual review of test workload, manual, semi-automated, and automated is necessary. The location of peripheral devices is dependent on the location of test sites and major instruments. General laboratory data processing policy influences the total number of such devices to be installed.

It is important to clearly identify the number and type of telephone or other telecommunication devices to be installed in the laboratory. Today prewiring is almost an essential feature as changes made after installation are often expensive.

The Data Base—Number of Personnel

1. Total (FTE–Glossary)
2. Peak number
   - *total*
   - *section*

In general, knowledge of the total number of personnel employed in the laboratory is not of great use in the planning process nor is the total FTE count of great value. What is important, however, is a plan outlining the maximum work force expected to be present in any given work station at routine and other times. These data are closely related to the test workload information and that gathered from a review of the instrumentation configuration plan.

In conclusion, the collection of useful laboratory data should be a relatively simple procedure. It is important to be aware of the changes which have occurred in laboratory practice, to understand how important proper interpretation of the data base is to the functional plan, and the necessity to relate many separate data items to achieve this level of interpretation.

The Data Base—A National Survey

Appendix E contains the data from a survey of 201 laboratories. These data include an analysis of the demographics, working space, workload, and personnel of these laboratories. For comparative purposes in the planning process of construction or remodeling, the reader will find the data useful. These data show the differences and similarities that exist between laboratories in a variety of institutional sizes and settings. Pathologists will find good examples of which data to gather in the planning process. Architects will find the data useful in orienting themselves to the various people, production, and space factors that impact on medical laboratory design. This survey represents one of the major highlights of this book and the reader is encouraged to peruse it carefully.

CONSTRAINTS IN PLANNING AND DESIGN 10

ONE OF THE MOST SIGNIFICANT PROBLEMS that interferes with the completion of a satisfactory design solution may be found within the overall building plan.

Physical Constraints: *Building*

When planning a facility within an existing structure the limitation is related more frequently to shape and location rather than work area. Shape is certainly more important than size and every effort must be made to determine that the final allotted work areas are of proper functional design. A reduction in square-foot allotment may be desirable to provide such a functional space. Redesign within an existing building may require the separation of work areas to separate floors. Before accepting such a possibility, functional activity and cost-effective operation should be considered. A collection or accessioning area at some distance from the most active processing unit may require additional staff merely for the transport of specimens. With large work areas, the planner must be prepared to deal with problems related only to the distance from the furthest point in the laboratory to the exit.

Modern design often provides for a laboratory with a minimum of non-supporting walls. This achievement may be difficult within an old building but should always be attempted. Additional problems which may be met are those connected with lighting, fire escape routing, and patient access.

Problems found within the building of old design also may be encountered with new construction. Frequently, the shape of the laboratory is determined by facilities located on floors above or below the work area. Outside building design in which windows are placed for esthetic reasons may pose a problem. Care should be taken with window design as broad glass areas are more detrimental than useful. Often the view provides little pleasure to busy staff, and problems created by excessive heat absorption may be serious. Vertical grid design and mechanical services are general building features which may interfere initially with the planning process. Early knowledge of the location of ducts and load-bearing walls is helpful in determining a reasonable solution. Care should be taken in the placement of mechanical facilities away from areas which are planned for future expansion.

Physical Constraints: *Site*

Problems associated with the site tend to be minimal with existing structures unless the laboratory facility is required to occupy a structure physically remote from the main building.

New construction may be planned for an area on the site which poses a problem for the laboratory. Occasionally, space is limited between an existing building and an existing roadway or some other physical impediment. Early attention to such a situation helps in the solution of the design problem. Special attention should always be paid to the location, design, and shading of windows if site selection suggests excessive heat exposure.

Intra-institutional Policies

The final laboratory design often is affected by general hospital administrative policies which apply to the complete building project. While frequently such decisions are of no serious consequence, at other times it is essential that details be fully understood before the laboratory plan is completed. These would include the following:

1. Mechanical and communication systems

2. Standard floor finishes

3. Standard casework for office and reception areas

Materials management policy is an influence on the decision to provide a central complete storage function within the laboratory using staff and space, or a top-up system with supplies moved to the site by other hospital personnel.

If an institutional policy requires preadmission screening, the laboratory plan requires that collection facilities are placed adjacent to the admitting area of the hospital.

Outpatient services such as parking should be considered if an institutional goal is the provision of a complete community health program. The laboratory should reflect general planning with the creation of a bright, colorful, and esthetically pleasant place in which to work. Applied economics are essential in the modern workplace and are illustrated by the use of proper chair design and variable height of work surfaces. Perhaps the most important aspect of this area of concern is that of representation. The laboratory director must strive for adequate membership on the general planning committee, or gain assurance that important institutional policy is communicated directly to the laboratory staff. Attention to the laboratory plan alone is not sufficient. A regular review of the complete planning project provides an opportunity to identify difficulties which may be impossible to change unless spotted early in the process.

Personnel

The success of any planning process depends to a large degree on the presence of interested and capable laboratory staff members. The director is responsible for appointing a planning group representative for the several sections within the laboratory. Sometimes the most senior member of this section is not the most desirable person due to lack of interest or confidence in the process. Seniority or scientific skill are not the essential qualities but rather an interest and ability to work well with others. It is essential that every effort be made to ensure continuity so that important design features are not changed radically to meet a personal need.

66 . . . The success of any planning process depends to a large degree on the presence of interested and capable laboratory staff members. 99

Philosophy

As in most endeavors, the planning process should begin with confidence. Laboratory directors and members of the planning team must remind themselves that the full knowledge of laboratory medicine lies within their group. It is their responsibility to communicate needs clearly and promptly to hospital planners and architects, and not to assume that these individuals understand the complexities of laboratory operation. There is no place in the process for the delegation of medical or technical functions to others. This is perhaps the most common error and usually leads to serious problems. Confidence then, that laboratory staff, and no others, carry the final responsibility for the design is clear.

Confidence in staff and the planning process must be accompanied by the development of strategies aimed at obtaining the best possible location for the laboratory and adequate spatial arrangements. Evidence must be gathered to show that existing formulae that relate laboratory square footage to beds, workload units, or staff are totally unreliable. Only on completion of the initial planning steps will a reasonable estimate of laboratory size be possible. Such strategies may involve regular contact with the hospital administrator, senior members of the medical staff, and even perhaps members of the governing body of the institution. In developing and implementing these strategies, confidence and knowledge need the support of tact and other good interpersonal communication skills. The possession of these characteristics makes it possible to deal with changes in the overall master plan or in the major goals and objectives of the institution within which the laboratory is to be located.

Institution Types

Regardless of the type of institution involved, the planning process remains the same. An understanding of the relative involvement of state, municipal, or regional officials is necessary as well as any special restraints under which the planners are working. Some institutions of a community nature may require complete community services; others may wish to refer much to a secondary site; and still others may be of such a specialized nature that most work is of the referral type.

PROJECT FINANCING 11

IN CONSIDERING THE DEVELOPMENT of a new, renovated, or expanded laboratory, few aspects of the project are more important than the capital financing. Undoubtedly, the financial considerations of a construction program can pose some of the most perplexing problems of a new project. For this reason, a number of general principles should be kept in mind.

One of the initial considerations in the planning process should be the determination of the financial feasibility of a project. If this factor is not clearly evaluated at the earliest stages of planning, the project can be impaired severely. Without it, planners are unable to define the scope of the project, there is ongoing uncertainty as to the availability and source of funds, and opportunities for cost-containment may be lost.

Second, outside financial assistance should be sought as early as possible. Seldom does an organization have sufficient staff to plan and construct a facility; likewise, it seldom has adequate staff to properly develop and execute appropriate financing. Just as there are costs associated with building planning and design, there are costs associated with financing.

Third, trustees and management should work closely together to assure that the financial stability of the institution is not impaired by the decisions they make. Whether the organization incurs long-term debt, expends surplus funds, raises funds through philanthropic sources, or receives some sort of grant assistance, the financial structure of the organization is affected. Thus, the impact of their decision should be considered carefully, and the long-term viability of the institution protected.

Financing Overview

Throughout much of the history of the American health care system, capital financing was provided by philanthropic donations. In the late 1940s, there was a major shift in health care capital financing when Congress passed what has become known as the Hill-Burton Act. With this act, major capital needs of new and existing health care facilities were met. This legislation signaled the emergence of a large number of new or expanded hospitals and marked the decline in need for philanthropic donations and the health care industry's dependence on them.

In the mid-1960s, another major change occurred in capital formation. The government shifted its capitalization effort from direct grants under Hill-Burton to recognition and payment of interest and depreciation expense under the Social Security Act that created Medicare.

Also in the mid-1960s, more hospitals took a look at their internal operations as a source of capital. Until this time, many hospitals operated on a pure nonprofit basis. They did not attempt to recover the cost of capital or to generate and fund excess revenues for future capital needs. At this time, operating philosophies began to change and organizations began to structure their financial management to generate sufficient surpluses to fund existing or future capital needs. Net income placed in reserve has become a significant source of capital.

With the evolution of financial philosophy and the development of profit generating strategies, a new form of capital appeared—investment capital. The emergence of for-profit companies has occurred within our generation and the impact they will have on capital formation in both the for-profit and nonprofit sector is still unknown. It is known, however, that these companies have been extremely successful in raising needed capital.

With the rapid escalation of cost, the technological advancements seen in the past two decades, and the seemingly increasing demand by consumers, the sources of capital already mentioned have not been sufficient to meet capital needs. As a result, there has been a movement toward borrowed capital. This creates a set of fiscal circumstances and considerations far different than the use of donations, funded reserves, direct government aid, and investment capital.

Permanent Capital

Permanent capital is available for use at any time an organization wants it with few conditions attached. However, debt financing is available only for a given period of time, must be repaid, and incurs an interest expense. Despite the opposite meanings of the terms, it is safe to say that the level of permanent capital often determines the availability of debt financing. Major sources of permanent capital are excess income; grants from federal, state, and private groups; and philanthropic contributions.

Excess income has become a major source of permanent capital. With the proper mix of private-pay, privately insured, and government-insured patients, excess income over expenses provides for significant capital funding. Generally speaking, this has worked well for hospitals in the last 20 years. Unfortunately, the future of this source is uncertain.

With soaring costs, more patients covered by cost-based federal programs, and more and more private insurance companies switching to cost-based reimbursement, the future of excess income as a source of permanent capital is in jeopardy. Because of this, the organization's permanent capital must be protected. Ways to preserve permanent capital through alternative financing methods should be explored, and efforts should be made to expand permanent capital through alternative sources of income. Federal, state, and private assistance programs have many shortcomings because they provide too little capital, and often are sporadic and expensive to apply for. Although many disadvantages are associated with these sources of funds, they should not be overlooked. They do represent sources of permanent capital and may encourage other sources of funds including donations and debt financing. These sources are varied and should be explored in the earliest stages of the project.

For many years, philanthropic donations supplied a large part of the capital needs of hospitals. Although these donations are at an all-time high, the percent of capital need met by such sources is no longer as significant as it was in the past. Capital needs have far exceeded the funds available through donations. Today, contributed funds are evidence of community support for an institution or a special project, and are extremely important as other sources of funds are sought. They provide matching funds for grants, supplemental amounts needed when going after debt financing, and ease the passage through regulatory bodies when need review is held.

Fund raising must be handled professionally with staff and money committed to the effort. Several groups within the hospital itself can be lucrative sources of philanthropy. If an employer has been successful at instilling loyalty and pride in the institution, employees should be receptive to the opportunity of showing their appreciation in return.

A second internal group which should be considered is the medical staff. In most cases, this group has a larger per capita income of any internal group solicited. In dealing with this body, several factors should be considered. These include timing, promotion of a project which they support, and some indication by the hospital of how much is expected from them.

Another internal group to consider is the volunteers or auxiliary. The potential for volunteer-generated funds is significant if properly managed. It should be clear that volunteer groups within the hospital can serve as more than social outlets. When given specific and reasonable goals, there is little reason to doubt the goal can be achieved.

Another internal area often overlooked in fundraising efforts is former patients. Generally, a patient leaves the hospital deeply grateful for his care, has not directly paid anything for his care, and sometimes wishes to show his appreciation. In as much as the hospital already has mailing information, the patient is a good source for a direct-mail campaign.

One last internal group to consider is the multitude of visitors that come to the hospital. Like patients, they too may wish to express their appreciation.

Having reviewed publics which exist within the hospital, several groups should be considered outside the hospital. First, the hospital should have a well-organized and active foundation. This organization can serve as a depository for hospital capital funds and shelter these funds against cost reimbursement formulae requiring depletion of such reserves. This organization also can serve as an active fundraising entity. In addition to its fundraising potential, separately incorporated foundations also are capable of borrowing money. Advantages of such an organization should be carefully explored in developing long-term capital development.

Local industry and organized labor usually are anxious to contribute to specific hospital fund drives. These organizations should be approached when specific identifiable projects are being considered.

Lastly, efforts should be made to develop special projects with the help of charity groups or foundations. These groups often are willing to fund projects related to their areas of interest.

Debt Financing

With the forces of capital finance changing within the health care field, there is a growing movement to debt financing. Some argue that debt financing should be the last alternative, and that all of an organization's permanent capital should be expended before debt is incurred. Arguments for and against debt financing will not be resolved in this publication. Debt financing will be considered as an option for capital financing.

There are basically two forms of debt financing—direct and indirect financing. Direct financing can be broken down into two categories which include bond financing and mortgage financing. The components of the various options available in these areas are reviewed below.

Tax-exempt bond financing has gained tremendous popularity in recent years. Earnings realized by bond holders are tax-exempt, and because of this, bonds are often issued at a rate of return significantly below similar quality issues. These bonds can be issued by state or municipal authorities, a city or county, or directly by a nonprofit corporation.

This method of financing allows one of the highest ratios of financing—often up to 100 percent. In addition, expenses incurred in developing the bond issue, interest expense during construction, and refinancing of existing debt can be included in the financial amount. Maturity dates of this form of financing can range up to 40 years and allow reduced annual debt service.

One should be cognizant that this form of financing may lead to a need for increased borrowing as a result of financing expenses, legal and printing costs, bond reserve fund, and capitalized interest during construction. Because of the complexity of this method the processing time may be longer than other alternatives.

Public taxable bonds are an option little used today because of alternative sources of financing. This method once was used widely and involved an investment banking firm or institutional bond house underwriting the loan and distributing the bonds to the public. Taxable bonds usually provide less than 60 percent of the financing needed and are issued for relatively short periods of time—15 to 20 years. This often requires refinancing of the unamortized balance.

FHA issued mortgages are available through the FHA 242 Mortgage Insurance Program. This program was developed to encourage the use of private institutional funds in health facilities development. It gives an added sense of security to investors which in turn allows the borrower to secure financing at a lower cost. The program allows high ratio financing, up to 90 percent, and can be combined with other sources of funds.

Private placement is a complicated method of debt financing requiring a high degree of expertise. The method involves the use of institutional lenders with taxable offerings which may include conventional mortgages, secured or unsecured notes, term loans with banks, and construction loans. The lenders may include pension funds, mutual funds, mutual savings banks, life insurance companies, savings and loan associations, and real-estate trusts. This method of financing is one of the quickest means of raising capital. However, the ratio of financing is lower than other methods, usually 50 percent or less, necessitating the need for alternative capital. In addition, restrictions placed on these securities might be stringent and may include shorter term, limited prepayment provisions, and higher interest rates.

Indirect financing involves the use of various lease arrangements. Lease financing usually covers a period of 20 to 30 years. The terms vary depending on the accounting advantages one hopes to achieve. There are a number of advantages to lease financing. These include off-balance sheet financing, advantageous rates as a result of tax benefits realized by the lessor, and alternative source financing which leaves more traditional sources unused in 100 percent financing. Disadvantages include the loss of tax incentives that are available to the lessee, loss of residual property value at the end of the lease, and lack of flexibility in use of the property.

Lease arrangements are not commonly used techniques for construction or renovation, but may prove to be extremely helpful in the acquisition of capital equipment.

Conclusion

There is no one single method of capital financing that is best. Instead, a selection of alternatives are available which must be judged in view of each institution's capital management strategy.

The capital management strategy should take into consideration how much capital is needed. Of this amount, how much is currently available, and how much is needed from outside sources.

One also must consider when capital is needed. In many cases, construction is ready to begin before proper financing is arranged, leading to costly delays and hastily arranged and sometimes inappropriate financing.

Small project financing also should be done in a manner that does not inhibit or affect adversely future capital financing by the institution as a whole. Of particular concern is the ability to pay back early, refinance, and/or incur additional financing.

" . . . There is no one single method of capital financing that is best. Instead, a selection of alternatives are available which must be judged in view of each institution's capital management strategy."

110

Careful analysis should be made of the cost of financing capital. As shown previously, there is a wide range of cost associated with capital financing and the institution should take advantage of the most convenient source in view of institutional needs.

Lastly, as mentioned in the beginning, outside assistance should be sought any time major capital expenditures are anticipated, particularly if extended financing is used. Investment in such expertise is money well spent.

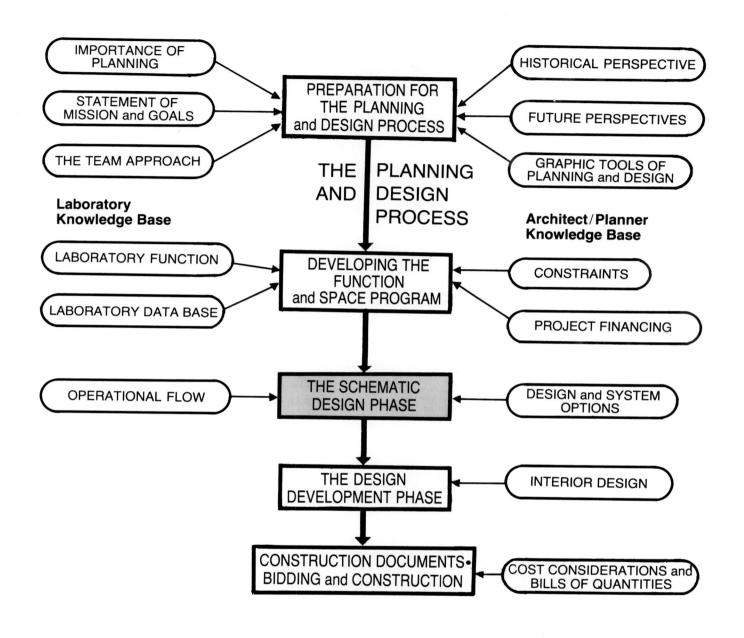

IMPORTANCE OF PLANNING

STATEMENT OF MISSION and GOALS

THE TEAM APPROACH

PREPARATION FOR THE PLANNING and DESIGN PROCESS

HISTORICAL PERSPECTIVE

FUTURE PERSPECTIVES

GRAPHIC TOOLS OF PLANNING and DESIGN

THE PLANNING
AND DESIGN
PROCESS

Laboratory Knowledge Base

Architect/Planner Knowledge Base

LABORATORY FUNCTION

LABORATORY DATA BASE

DEVELOPING THE FUNCTION and SPACE PROGRAM

CONSTRAINTS

PROJECT FINANCING

OPERATIONAL FLOW

THE SCHEMATIC DESIGN PHASE

DESIGN and SYSTEM OPTIONS

THE DESIGN DEVELOPMENT PHASE

INTERIOR DESIGN

CONSTRUCTION DOCUMENTS• BIDDING and CONSTRUCTION

COST CONSIDERATIONS and BILLS OF QUANTITIES

Part III
THE SCHEMATIC DESIGN PHASE

SCHEMATIC DESIGN 12

THE SCHEMATIC DESIGN PHASE is the strongest interactive phase between the owner and the architect. During this phase all the information developed during the programming, bubble, and block diagram phases are integrated into the design which, for the first time, begins to take the form of a building. At this time, additional factors are considered as the design evolves. The layout now is influenced by life safety codes, building construction requirements such as structural grids, mechanical chases, and spaces for equipment—mechanical and electrical, means of circulation of both intradepartment and interdepartment including stairs, elevators, main circulation corridors, and other systems.

Before this stage, any number of people may have been involved in the development of documents. Probably, the hospital planner or pathologist has been responsible for developing the bulk of documents up to this point. However, at this stage an architect should be involved. The project team continues to grow through this stage. It should consist of a laboratory representative, architect, design engineers (usually included as part of the architect's basic services), and a hospital or institutional representative, if applicable.

If the size of the project warrants it, the general contractor or construction manager may be part of the team for providing value engineering. Alternately, this information can be provided by the architect or cost estimator. The process of value engineering at an early design stage allows several alternative systems to be evaluated, both in terms of cost and performance. A typical example is the structural system. After the initial floor plan sketches are complete and a tentative structural grid is laid out, several alternative structural systems may be proposed and evaluated. A structural steel grid versus a poured-in-place concrete framework versus a precast concrete framework, or perhaps even a combination of bearing walls and structural spanning members may be considered. They should be evaluated from the standpoint of cost of materials, erection procedures and technique, additional treatments which may be necessary such as fireproofing, length of erection time, and availability of materials in the location

115

being planned. Additionally, a construction manager or general contractor may be able to assist in the coordination of the various disciplines.

Clear communication between the architect and the laboratory representative is most important during the schematic design period. During this stage, a number of final decisions are made on a broad variety of levels. The specific size, layout, location, and physical relationship to adjacent spaces are determined for all functional elements in the laboratory. Decisions involving abstract ideas such as flexibility, esthetic quality of the environment, function and flow, between sections and communications are specifically laid out and determined during this stage. For this reason, all members of the project team must concentrate their efforts and availability to ensure that data and concepts developed during the previous stages are realized in the design. Furthermore, assumptions made previously are now tested and confirmed.

Frequently, difficulties are encountered in this stage due to the inability of the various professionals involved to adequately communicate with each other. The laboratory representative may not be used to dealing with the graphic tools of the architect (the drawings). It is therefore incumbent on the architect to develop drawings which are most clearly readable and comprehensible to the layman. As the schematic design progresses, it is the architect's responsibility to ensure that the design, as represented by the schematic drawings, is understood by the user. Devices such as the graphic representation of furniture, equipment, and perhaps people, make the drawings more intelligible and lend scale to the design.

The issue of scale is perhaps the greatest source of misunderstanding during this stage and eventually in the actual construction of the building. While the architect may make a great effort during the entire design process to try and relate the actual size of the space in dimension, or even a combination of dimensions, it is not unusual for a user to walk into the final space and say that it is smaller than anticipated. Commonly, laboratory personnel feel that the final plan has no relationship to the drawings prepared. Every effort must be made to ensure that all parties involved understand the drawings during this stage.

Early in the schematic phase, other types of building systems may be considered to provide some of the functional requirements which have been identified in earlier stages. A number of systems for transportation of people and materials are available. For instance, stairs, elevators, escalators, ramps, pneumatic tube systems, cart lifts, automated cart systems, and robotics are

> " . . . Clear communication between the architect and the laboratory representative is most important during the schematic design period. "

116

available and in use in the laboratory today. The quality and performance of all these systems should be considered as possible solutions to the performance requirements specified in the early planning and design efforts. The relative cost of these systems also must be included at this time. Selection of some of these systems are obvious while others require much more detailed thought. The project team finds this stage of design as a time of creating, testing, and revising the design. It is important that everyone's continued effort be maintained to ensure that the work done to this point is realized in the design of the building.

Concepts such as flexibility must be kept in mind. It must be understood that the architect is developing a specific layout which cannot be modified easily at the end of the schematic stage. However, it is not unusual for the period between the end of schematic design and the actual occupancy of the finished product to be a number of years. This is particularly true in a project in which a number of construction phases occur in order to ensure that operations are maintained during construction or renovation of the new facilities. Therefore, the notion of flexibility is an important concept to be maintained in the design. Assumptions and decisions made during the programming and design phase may be somewhat altered or even altogether invalidated during the period of construction. Also, decisions and assumptions can and will change after occupancy of the new facility. For these reasons, it continues to be important to design a space which is not so customized that changes cannot be accomplished with minimum disruption and modification to the laboratory design.

Elements which contribute to the flexibility or inflexibility of the laboratory include such components as structural columns, fixed partitions, exterior walls, mechanical shafts, water supply, drainage systems, and other utilities. While it is conceivable that all of these elements could be totally flexible, it is generally cost prohibitive to provide these in such a manner. A more reasonable and practical approach may be to limit the use of these elements where feasible. However, the most effective way to provide flexibility is simply to locate the fixed items in areas where flexibility is least necessary. In areas where the most changes are likely to occur, provide the least number of fixed elements. This is possible by keeping the number of laboratory functions enclosed in fixed partitions to an absolute minimum. Generally, this may be limited to areas which are hazardous to surrounding areas, require unusual isolation from other areas, or perhaps even require fireproof construction to enclose. However, areas which can be left open should be. This allows adjacent areas to expand into that space if necessary or allows that function itself to grow into adjacent spaces. Flexibility

117

also can be provided in the selection of equipment and casework. Systems that can be moved quickly will encourage the laboratory to continue to explore new layouts as conditions and understanding needs change and improve.

Perhaps the most useful attitude at this point is to realize that the entire design may require compromises from the ideal solution in almost every case. However, also realize that almost every situation in a person's daily work experience requires some compromise and yet effective environments exist all around us which allow us to accomplish the task at hand. With this in mind, it should be possible to proceed through the schematic design with sound and fundamental concepts for maintaining flexibility, yet still make the specific decisions which enable the planning and design process to proceed into construction and eventual occupancy. Remember that the objective is not to create a design; the objective is to create a building that is functional as a laboratory.

Before schematic design, and perhaps even in the initial stages of schematic design, the planning has been limited to two-dimensional design. During the schematic development, the design begins to take on three-dimensional characteristics. These include the height of the building, the number of stories, vertical relationships required by function or in response to site conditions such as a hilly site. As in the development of the two-dimensional plans, the schematic three-dimensional plans evolve through a series of progressive detailed designs. At first, only gross functional relationships are shown in a vertical manner. The floor to floor heights and general exterior massing of the buildings are studied. As structural systems and other engineering systems are developed, the dimensions required for these systems to perform begin to impact on the vertical relationships of the building. For instance, a structural beam has a required depth to span a specific distance. In addition, the mechanical duct work and other systems require space above the occupied floor level to provide the distribution required. Integration and coordination of all the systems is one of the most vital activities which must be undertaken throughout the schematic design phase and through construction and occupancy. It is incumbent on the project team leader and all of the team members to be aware of and responsive to the needs of the various disciplines which are now involved in the planning process.

Provisions for future expansion must be anticipated and accommodated at this point. If it is desirable to provide for some future vertical expansion of the building with additional floors, elements such as the foundations and structural grid must be designed in such a way to anticipate these future loads. In addition,

" . . . Perhaps the most useful attitude at this point is to realize that the entire design may require compromises from the ideal solution in almost every case."

118

it may be desirable to size the primary utilities to the building for these additional loads, thereby reducing the development costs and modifications required at the time expansion is undertaken. However, a price must be paid for all of this flexibility and a judgment made as to what is most likely versus what is perhaps a long-term notion of what future requirements are necessary. The purpose of providing for future expansion should be more than simply an expedient "just in case." It quickly becomes apparent that making provisions for unlimited growth also entails an unlimited budget.

The architect develops additional documents beyond the drawings during the schematic phase. An outline specification should be developed which describes in a narrative form types of utilities, systems, finishes, and other specific building characteristics. The outline specification's purpose is to give a broad description of the scope of the project and its detailed elements. It should indicate the quality of the systems desired with the backup of the schematic drawings to provide some notion of quantity. The schematic design phase involves more than one drawing and one review. As noted before, it is a time of constant interaction between the owner, user, and designer. The drawings are developed over a period of time and continue to explore relationships desired, alternatives which are available, and resolution of conflicts and problems. The scale at which the drawings are prepared may change during the schematic design to a larger scale in order that specific problems and solutions may be explored. Drawings at ⅛ in = 1 ft or even ¼ in = 1 ft are not uncommon, and in fact, are useful for this stage of drawings. At a larger scale, detailed relationships and sizes can be more accurately represented and studied. At ¹⁄₁₆ in = 1 ft it is most common for only single-line walls and openings to be shown. At a larger ⅛ in = 1 ft it is possible to show wall thicknesses, door swings, some equipment and casework layouts and other requirements in a more detailed manner. At ¼ in = 1 ft it is possible to accurately show all elements of laboratory furniture and equipment and even details of utility distribution. More drawing effort is required and more detail shown with a larger scale. It is therefore important to select a scale at which only the appropriate detail is required and thereby spend no more time than is necessary in preparing each drawing.

Depending on the needs of the particular project, the level of detail which is developed during the schematic design period varies. It may be adequate to simply develop single-line documents (¹⁄₁₆ in = 1 ft) for a particular project during the schematic phase. However, in other circumstances, it may be necessary to fully develop each of the spaces showing all bench work, equipment, door swings, plumbing fixtures, and all the other items anticipated. The latter is, however, the exception as this detail is usually developed during the design development phase.

The schematic design phase ends with a formal review and approval process. As stated before, it is most important that the documents developed during this phase be intelligible to all parties involved. However, more effort may be required including use of models and perspective drawings. These often may be in the form of rough working sketches.

The completed single-line drawings represent firm decisions with regard to the location of all fixed and major moveable equipment. It indicates that the rooms have been placed in proper relationship, that flow is as desired, that all spaces, rooms, and areas are the right shape and dimension, and that openings to these areas are properly placed and provisions adequately realized for future expansion and flexibility. All engineering systems have been initially designed and selected. All casework has been initially laid out and types of systems evaluated. Assumptions made during the programming and block diagramming phase have been tested, confirmed, or modified. This may include zoning approval, Department of Health approval, institutional review and approval such as the Board of Directors or county agency approval.

Also, at the completion of the schematic phase, a more accurate probable construction cost may be developed. As this probable construction cost is developed, it may be necessary or possible to modify the schematics developed. It may be necessary to reduce the cost of the project proposed, or additional scope may be added to the project to use more fully the project budget. In any case, the project team is well advised to proceed only after the cost estimates have been completed on this phase. As with all estimates, the more accurate the information used in developing it, the more reliable the figure is.

Other Considerations of Schematic Design

Equipment Planning

An integral facet of the schematic design phase is equipment planning. The laboratory, as much as any type of facility and more than most, has a complex array of equipment ranging from items such as bulky refrigerators to the most sensitive and delicate bench top instruments. Through the planning and design process, equipment planning must be integrated with other needs to identify both the need for and types of equipment. This planning should include an evaluation of existing equipment to be reused and a listing of new equipment to be purchased.

In the early stages of the project, the equipment planning effort should concentrate on determining the scope of equipment to be reused versus items to be purchased. A preliminary budget should be established and factored in with the other project costs. In addition, information on major items of equipment which impact on the preliminary design of the architect and the engineers must be compiled and distributed so that the loads and sizes may be identified and tested against the space allocation program. This information also tells the architect and engineer of any special conditions which have to be addressed in design, such as unusual weight loads, heavy heat loads, and special ventilation, and service or power requirements.

Equipment is one of the most significant factors in contemporary laboratory planning and design. Trends toward more instrumentation and automation require that the entire project team be cognizant of the impact this has on design.

Engineering Systems

Either concurrently with or following the initial layouts of spaces and rooms, the engineering systems also should be schematically developed. These include structural, mechanical, plumbing, and electrical systems. The structural grid must be determined and alternative structural systems analyzed. The mechanical requirements and environmental conditions should be analyzed initially and systems for providing these conditions developed. Similarly, the plumbing and electrical systems in terms of loads, quality, and layout also should be considered. It is important at this stage to have available for the engineers the space program, Room Data Sheets, a major equipment schedule, and any other information developed during the earlier stages so that the initial loads and performance requirements can be understood and analyzed by the design engineers. As with most other elements in the design, a number of options may be available in the selection and configuration of all these systems. To the architect, the development of these systems requires integrating the space requirements of each of these systems with the space requirements of the laboratory functions. For example, the structural system undoubtedly has columns or bearing walls that require certain minimum dimensions. The mechanical systems may require risers or duct work, equipment rooms for air handling units, and electrical equipment. All of these systems must be incorporated into the space assignments allocated during the schematic design in order for the laboratory planning to be converted into a working environment.

Site Analysis

At this point, the location of the building on a site also must be developed in much the same manner as the initial layouts of the interior spaces. The site constraints first must be identified and then options for dealing with the constraints as well as the functional requirements must be explored in much the same manner in which interior space has been developed. Typical constraints include zoning codes for that particular building. A zoning code may specify whether a laboratory may be built on a particular site. It usually also determines setbacks from property lines which must be maintained, number of parking spaces, types and numbers of loading facilities for service vehicles and trash removal, landscaping, site development specifications, and other requirements. Availability of utilities to the proposed new construction also must be analyzed and accounted for at the time that the site is selected. If there is an option in choosing a site, it is desirable to limit the development costs incurred in building the new facility by having utilities required available either on site or nearby. Utilities such as water service, electricity, sewer systems and energy sources must be considered. If any of these are not available, they have to be developed, usually at the owner's expense. For instance, if a sewer is not available at the site, it may be necessary to develop an on-site package system. These can be costly and may rule out a particular site or make the project infeasible. Obviously, it is important that these considerations be identified and resolved before any unnecessary effort in the planning and design stage proceeds.

LABORATORY OPERATIONAL FLOW 13

PROGRAMMING AND ARRANGING SPACE AND EQUIPMENT in the clinical laboratory is to be preceded by a thorough understanding of the functions to be accomplished, and of the various flows that are part of those functions. In this chapter the concept of operational flow for generalized laboratory functions is discussed. Specific functions of the various laboratory sections are covered in chapter 8. The more generalized functions of test ordering, specimen collection, specimen organization and distribution, testing, result reporting, and materials management are included here. These functions are common to all laboratory sections in one form or another. The figures in this chapter should serve to illustrate the impact of function and flow on laboratory design. This is a most critical concept for good design and one that should be understood thoroughly.

Flow—Kinds of Flow

The term *flow* is used here in the technical sense of spatial flow of people, materials, and informational data. The laboratory is much like a highly specialized manufacturing facility. Spatial relationships are critical to efficient movement of material and personnel use. It is the planner's responsibility to identify the flows that accompany particular functions in a specific case, and incorporate those flows into the spatial design. There is great variation in flow from laboratory to laboratory. A checklist of flows to be considered is shown in the following chart. The list is not necessarily complete but of sufficient scope to impart to the reader the importance of understanding the flow concept.

In principle, each flow component pairs with each of the function components to produce a larger set of flow-function pairs; however, some paired sets of flow and function are more important than others; e.g., report flow is much more significant to the reporting function than to the test ordering func-

" . . . It is the planner's responsibility to identify the flows that accompany particular functions in a specific case, and incorporate those flows into the design."

tion. We begin with orders, and trace the significance of flow to each of the major functions.

Table 13.1 Function and Flow Chart

FUNCTION	ORDERS	ROU SPEC	EMR SPEC	REPORTS	PEOPLE	MATERIAL	BLOOD
TEST ORDERING	X		X				
SPEC. COLLECTION		X	X		X		
ORGANIZ and DISTRIB.			X		X		X
TESTING		X			X		
RESULT REPORTING				X	X		
MATERIALS MANAGEMENT		X			X	X	

Orders—Flow of Orders in Test Ordering

Test ordering for inpatients and outpatients is normally initiated from the patient service unit, either as a requisition form or as an entry into a computerized ordering system. When the manually generated requisitions are delivered to the laboratory, whether by messenger or by pneumatic tube carrier, they should be received at a clerical station established for this purpose. Computer entry systems require a small station with printer for receiving orders (Fig. 13.1).

One copy of the test requisition usually remains in the laboratory after the test is completed, and provision should be made to store these forms; either within the spatial confines of the order receiving station, or at a separate file area. The amount of space required for storing requisitions depends on the format of the form, the number of years of orders to be kept on active file, and the size of the laboratory's patient load. For example, if the form is 8½ in × 11 in and five years of active orders are to be retained within the laboratory, and the workload is 30,000 orders per year, space and storage equipment for 150,000 or-

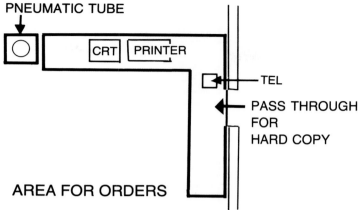

PNEUMATIC TUBE

CRT PRINTER

TEL

PASS THROUGH
FOR
HARD COPY

AREA FOR ORDERS

Fig. 13.1

Example of a space for receiving test orders via pneumatic tube, computer system, or hand delivery.

ders, each 8½ in × 11 in, must be provided. At a file packing density of 100 orders per inch, 1,500 linear inches of file space, or approximately ten file cabinets three feet deep by four drawers high, are required.

Orders—Flow of Orders in Other Functions

The flow of the test order in all laboratory functions does not require accumulation beyond a daily workload. Exceptions to this are those orders that cannot be completed in one day, e.g., microbiology orders or orders referred to outside laboratories. Each functional component of the laboratory should have a small temporary place to hold orders in process.

Routine Specimens—Flow of Routine Specimens in Specimen Collection

Routine specimens should be received in the laboratory at a central specimen receiving station or accessioning area, whether the specimens are brought in by the phlebotomists, collected by laboratory staff from outpatients, mailed in, received from messengers, or by other means (Fig. 13.2). The identification of the specimen by an appropriate ID number requires a clerical station, which can be the same station that receives test orders. The size of this station depends primarily on the laboratory workload. For example, if one clerk can receive and organize specimens at the rate of four per minute (not allowing for rest, breaks, and other nonproductive activities), then a station operating at 75 percent overall productivity can handle 180 specimens per hour. Only large lab-

125

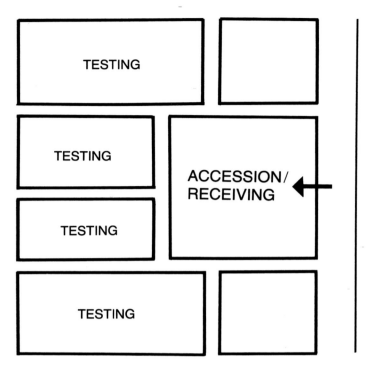

Fig. 13.2

Relationship of specimen receiving to testing is one of a central receiving space with access to each of the major testing spaces.

oratories can justify an entire station dedicated to this function, and in most cases other functions (e.g., appointments) can be combined at this station.

This station also can be responsible for dispatching phlebotomists to collection assignments, and space should be provided for this purpose. Typical space requirements for phlebotomists include a work counter with space for each phlebotomist to assemble a tray with the necessary supplies and some short-term storage space for daily supplies (Fig. 13.3).

Routine Specimens—Flow of Routine Specimens in Specimen Organization and Distribution

In order to provide consistently rapid reporting, routine specimens should not accumulate to a degree greater than is necessary to match the workload with efficient equipment or persons doing each test. For example, if the glucose test load is 100 tests per day and a batch analyzer capable of ten samples

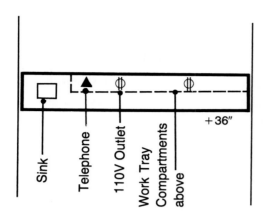

Fig. 13.3

Example of a space suitable for phlebotomists who work from a "base" station.

per 15-minute batch is performing the tests, one can plan to do about one batch every two to three hours, and in most cases a specimen need not wait more than two hours before being tested. Because the various testing stations are working in parallel, the specimen distribution function must be designed so that distribution does not limit the production capability of the laboratory. For example, assuming a peak workload arrival rate of 50 specimens every hour, the specimen distribution should be able to assign these specimens to the appropriate work station within the one hour available. When specimens are divided to allow different tests from the same specimen (e.g., glucose and BUN from a serum specimen), even more distribution capability is needed. Specimen distribution should include any preparation of the sample, as well as the necessary clerical work to determine location of the specimen and the estimated test completion time. These requirements probably add up to a dual work station (one clerical position and one specimen handling position) for most laboratories, and perhaps a larger and multiple arrangement for the busy laboratory.

Routine Specimens—Flow of Routine Specimens in Testing

The flow of routine specimens through the various testing stations is the heart of the laboratory's productive capability. The choice of equipment and methodology sets the maximum rate at which testing can be done, and defines the rate at which the input functions (those that provide specimens to the testing stations) and the reporting station must operate in order for the laboratory to run smoothly and efficiently. Naturally, each testing component of the laboratory needs to have sufficient space, equipment, personnel, and materials to perform its daily workload, and the flow considerations here assume that the pathologist has already defined these needs to the designer. So far as the relation of routine specimens to the laboratory function goes, the designer's responsibility is to ensure that specimens can be received at and removed from the testing areas in an efficient manner. This generally means defining either unidirectional flow, or a radial flow pattern in which a central receiving and reporting area is functionally contiguous to testing areas. An undesirable case is one in which testing areas are adjacent to other testing areas in a linear pattern leading to a dead-end.

Routine Specimens—Flow of Routine Specimens in Materials Management

Specimens not saved after testing become part of the materials management process, i.e., the waste disposal portion of that management. Blood and urine samples should be decontaminated before disposal.

Some radioactive samples may have to be stored in shielded containers and held for disposal according to the rules of the Nuclear Regulatory Commission.

Contaminated samples that pose a danger to the laboratory and hospital staff, or the general public, should be decontaminated in a sterilizer provided for this purpose. This sterilizer may be located within the laboratory or in a central decontamination facility elsewhere in the hospital.

A soiled collection room should be provided within the laboratory, but close to the corridor access to the laboratory, for the flushing of liquid waste and the accumulation of solid waste for collection. Under no circumstances should this soiled collection room accumulate more than one day's waste.

STAT Specimens—Flow of STAT Specimens in Test Ordering

Special facilities or relationships may not be required within the laboratory for handling STAT orders. Should a STAT order be placed for a specimen that is already in the laboratory for a different purpose, the laboratory personnel must find that specimen and recategorize it. An orderly specimen distribution procedure makes this task a simple one.

STAT Specimens—Flow of STAT Specimen Collection

Whether certain phlebotomists are assigned to STAT collections or the most available phlebotomist is used, there is nothing inherently different for the design to collect such specimens.

STAT Specimens—Flow of STAT Specimens in Specimen Organization, Distribution, and Testing

There are several conceptual approaches for the distribution and testing of STATS, and one or another of these should be defined for the laboratory operation before design proceeds. Some laboratories test STATS in an area totally separate from that used for routine tests, even going so far as to locate satellite testing facilities. If there is a satellite laboratory, the designer has to consider it as a separate space with its own requirements for flow.

In other cases, STAT specimens come to the main or central laboratory, and the flow decision is either to use the same equipment for STAT testing that is used for routine testing, i.e., merely altering specimen positions to move the STAT specimen ahead of the routine specimen, or to dedicate separate equipment for STAT work. If the same equipment and facilities are being used, no additional spatial flow considerations are necessary; however, if different equipment or testing stations are being used, the designer should place the STAT facilities so that they bypass the main flow, and yet have as good access to the specimen receiving and reporting stations as the routine stations (Fig. 13.4).

Blood for Transfusions—Flow of Blood to and from Blood Bank

Whether blood is collected from donors or brought to the laboratory from outside sources, this blood should be identified, tested as necessary, and stored by the blood bank for later distribution.

Good access to the elevator-corridor system aids the blood bank in the rapid distribution of blood to the emergency and operating rooms and other areas.

Reports—Flow of Reports in Result Compilation

Reports either originate in the testing areas or are delivered to the laboratory with mail/messenger deliveries. In the former case, the reports move to the area programmed for report checking and dispatch. It is in this area that the report is checked for completeness and officially released from the laboratory. If

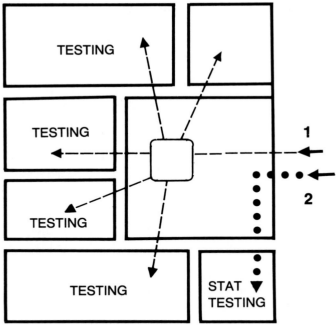

Fig. 13.4

Relationship of STAT testing to specimen receiving may have STAT specimens: **(1)** tested in the same spaces as routine specimens, or **(2)** diverted to a special STAT testing space.

the reporting form is different from the order form, as is often the case, another form of paper may be generated for storage (at a volume comparable to the volume of orders). Two solutions to the paper generation and storage problem deserve consideration: one solution is to place the test results on the same form that contains the order, and thus store only one piece of paper instead of two; another solution is to put test results into electronic form, store them on magnetic tape or disk, and print only the paper copy that leaves the laboratory. In the case of reports received from outside the laboratory, it is probably better to store the laboratory's hard copy of the report.

It is not difficult to imagine elaborate computerized configurations in which most test equipment (including outside equipment) reports directly into a central processor that controls all reporting functions. The disadvantage of such schemes is the interfacing. Standards are not sufficiently developed at this time to make interfacing a simple matter, and the pathologist may not want to constrain his choice of equipment in order to guarantee interfacing of data transfer. Interface costs can sometimes be high, and for economic reasons interfacing may be undesirable for low volume instruments.

130

People—General Movement of People

Since all the people who work in the laboratory require general access into, out of, and within the laboratory, free movement from space to space is essential. Fire and safety regulations regarding widths of corridors, protected accesses to exits, and dual exit paths from large spaces need to be obeyed. The designer should strive for a compromise between too much compartmentalization, which may increase productivity for some people while neglecting the general human interaction helpful to morale, and too much open space, which encourages distraction and lack of concentration. Glass partitions, which visually support a sense of group activity and yet reduce auditory distractions, are to be encouraged.

Salesmen should be discouraged from access to the laboratory. Conferences and demonstrations can be confined to spaces set aside for that purpose, either in general hospital space or in a laboratory conference room.

Likewise, physicians and residents who need to confer with the pathologist should be discouraged from entering the test areas, under the general rule that pathologists working in the test areas will contact them. In the discipline of anatomic pathology, it is desirable for medical staff and residents to have easy access to the pathologist's office or slide reading area.

People—Ambulatory Patients

The main classes of ambulatory patients who are served by the laboratory are:

- *Outpatients from whom specimens are to be obtained*
- *Blood donors*

Traditionally, most laboratories have provided waiting space and specimen collection facilities for outpatients. Although there is nothing inherently wrong with this practice, an examination of functional relationships may reveal that this is not a high priority need. The advantages of having such outpatient facilities contiguous to the laboratory are:

- *Being able to use a common staff*
- *Being able to move samples directly into the work flow*

The disadvantages are:

- *Having reception and waiting at the laboratory duplicate similar spaces already provided in the outpatient areas*
- *The need to accommodate outpatients may compromise other desirable design features, such as good staff or materials access*

131

If there is no assurance for efficient and reliable transport of samples into the laboratory, separate waiting and specimen collection areas contiguous to the laboratory should be provided.

To the extent that significant numbers of blood donors come to the hospital, it is probably better to provide space for this activity near the blood bank. Donations may occur in the evening under emergency conditions and there is a significant advantage using the same personnel to supervise the donation and perform the laboratory testing functions.

People—Flow of People in Specimen Collection

Phlebotomists and/or other staff who assist in specimen collection should have home stations near the periphery of the laboratory, with easy access to patients and the general access corridors. Patient spaces, including waiting spaces, venipuncture areas, toilets, etc., should likewise be located near the general access corridors and removed from the testing areas.

People—Flow of People in Specimen Organization and Distribution

The traffic of nurses and aides delivering specimens should not significantly mix with the flow of technologists or other staff distributing samples to the test area. One way to achieve this is to provide a pass-through opening for the handling of incoming specimens. Whether the specimens are distributed to the test areas by technologists who pick up the specimens, or by staff who work in the distribution areas, is a matter of choice. In a busy laboratory an aide who performs clerical tasks and delivers specimens may be justified. In either case, the staff distributing specimens within the laboratory should not have to enter the clerical and file space to pick up the specimens.

People—Flow of People in Test Areas

Since nearly all tests can be performed by one person using a few pieces of equipment, these are relatively static areas. Special attention should be given to easy and unobstructed movement from one equipment item to another (e.g., from automated analyzer to workbench) and to access to emergency safety equipment such as deluge showers, eye washes, and fire blankets. Specimen inflow and report outflow should occur from the outside margin of the module.

People—Flow of People in Reporting

Of course, reporting is the major output of the laboratory and a hard copy report is regarded as an essential document for the patient record. In the case of numeric test values, the report needs to be matched to the test order (or transcribed onto the test order) and this may be done by people in a clerical area, or by people in the test areas. The test values may be delivered from (or picked up from) the test areas, or generated on a printer located in the report area, but connected to the test equipment. Reports consisting of transcribed dictation may be generated in a designated portion of the reporting area, or in an area apart from the main laboratory.

People—Flow of People in Materials Management

The delivery of clean supplies and the removal of trash and reprocessible items should be performed by hospital staff, not laboratory staff, and the drop-off and pick-up points for these items should be on the periphery of the laboratory. Soiled collection, particularly, should be apart from the sample flow pattern, the report flow pattern, and the patient flow pattern. Clean supply delivery may be made via a central reception area; however, it is preferable that there be a separate entrance into the laboratory for this purpose. Rooms with two doors, one to the access corridor and one to the laboratory, are ideal for defining common access while separating the flow of people (Fig. 13.5).

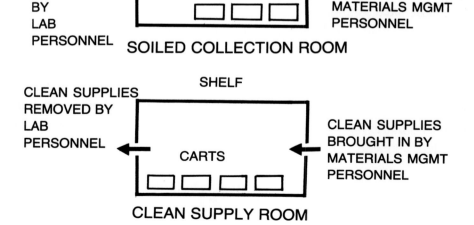

Fig. 13.5

Examples of clean and soiled holding rooms with dual access, one for materials management personnel and one for laboratory personnel.

Materials

Materials found in the laboratory may be classified as follows:

- *Chemicals and special laboratory supplies*
- *Glassware*
- *Paper and household supplies*
- *Waste*

Materials—Flow of Various Materials in Materials Management

Chemicals and special laboratory supplies that are consumed at a rapid rate and in high volume (e.g., vacutainers, prepared media) should be replenished from a bulk stores area, either one dedicated solely to laboratory use, or one that is a portion of the general bulk stores. Supplies unique to the laboratory should be stored in the laboratory, and other supplies in bulk stores. This area should be apart from, or peripheral to, the main laboratory space. Items consumed slowly and in low volumes can be accommodated within the storage space distributed about the laboratory.

If large volumes of glassware are washed and reused, a flow cycle to collect and distribute glassware items needs to be established. The glassware washing area should be peripheral to the test areas, but need not have access to the general corridors.

Paper and household supplies (e.g., paper towels, computer paper) should be kept in the laboratory in small quantities and replenished often (perhaps once a day) from the general bulk stores or central supply. Flammable materials in both bulk and small quantities need to be stored in special areas or cabinets designated as safe.

Waste should be collected or flushed away at frequent intervals; several collections daily are appropriate for nonhazardous waste. Organic solvents in small quantities may be flushed down drains with copious amounts of water. Contaminated wastes should be decontaminated in steam sterilizers; radioactive waste with long decay time may be stored in lead containers before removal from the laboratory. Radioactive waste with short decay time may be allowed to decay in lead containers and then be transferred to other containers.

DESIGN AND SYSTEM OPTIONS 14

CASEWORK OR LABORATORY FURNITURE DESIGN has been undergoing a tremendous evolution since the 1960s. Before the late 1960s and early 1970s casework was typically designed and manufactured in either wood or metal. It was often static or stationary in design with the usual Alberene stone, soap stone, or resin work surface. The finishes were either stain, varnish, or bonderized, baked enamel with brushed, chrome hardware, and it had to have the obligatory reagent shelf and water trough. Sinks were made of the same material as the work surface and were almost always located at the end of the bench. The workmanship was normally good to excellent and the casework was constructed to give many years of good service.

With the advent of the technical revolution in manufacturing and the introduction of automated laboratory equipment, coupled with changes in the health delivery system in general, the laboratory became a place for great activity and change. Automated tissue processors, single-channel analyzers and other automated equipment began to appear initially in the histology and chemistry sections followed shortly thereafter by similar automated equipment in hematology. Currently, microbiology is experiencing automated equipment growth.

In order to provide counter space, floor space, utilities and ventilation systems for the new equipment, it became evident that the traditional fixed or nonmoveable casework could not meet the demands for change or flexibility. Although many hospital planners believe new techniques, procedures, equipment, and space requirements for today's hospitals change constantly, no one area has been affected more radically than the laboratory.

To meet this challenge, individuals began to experiment with various forms of flexible or demountable casework in order to allow change or modification within the laboratory quickly, with minimum inconveniences at a low cost. A wooden prototype casework system was developed that addressed most of these requirements and eventually was recognized by the American casework industry and improved in design, quality, and flexibility. The original system was limited in the variety of casework components but had some unique mechanical and electrical features.

Presently, laboratory casework falls within the following three basic categories:

1. *Fixed casework* is nonmoveable, floor mounted with the work surfaces at a pre-established height from the floor for performing specific stand-up or sit-down tasks. The system does not allow the user the ability to raise or lower the work surface, interchange drawers, base cabinets, or wall cabinets.

2. *Modified casework* can be mounted to a utility chase or a wall rail and although the work surface is fixed, the base cabinets can be suspended under it or moved into a different configuration with the use of a small dolly. Wall cabinets are usually at a fixed height and are not moveable. There are systems which have moveable base cabinets mounted on casters which roll under a fixed work surface.

3. *Flexible or moveable casework systems* offer an unlimited ability to completely change a work station or the entire laboratory arrangement within certain limitations. The work surfaces can be raised, lowered, deleted, or added. Drawers, cabinets, files, shelves, or knee holes can be located as desired and moved with minimum effort. There are a variety of systems which allow the users to hang overhead cabinets, shelves, chalkboards, or tackboards at their discretion and there is an accessible service chase which offers ready access to utilities. The use of these systems allows the user to make minor modifications routinely and major changes quickly without the necessity of demolishing walls in order to expand an area or to access the utilities (Fig. 14.1). With easy access to the service chase, the process of renovation becomes less cumbersome, costly, and inconvenient. Often it can be accomplished without disruption to the daily laboratory operation.

In addition to fixed or moveable storage units, carts and transporters are available to enhance each system. Usually an acid-resistant plastic laminate

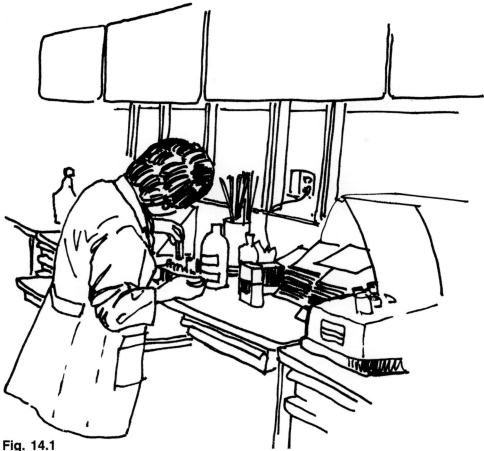

Fig. 14.1

Tackboard surfaces can be used to post notices, schedules, telephone numbers and act as a temporary divider between various divisions of the laboratory.

work surface is recommended but any work surface the user finds acceptable can be installed. Resin tops are recommended in hoods and are available from some of the flexible casework manufacturers who include hoods in their line of products.

Part of the flexible casework concept envisions some built-in obsolescence which allows the user to alter the various components of the system by drilling or screwing, discarding the components, and replacing them with the original. For example, a small pump or compressor may be attached to a work surface for a period of time and then discarded or replaced with a new one. A disposable cover is offered by one manufacturer that can be used in a staining area or heavy acid use area. When it becomes unsightly or damaged by the stains or acid, it can be discarded and replaced at less cost than a new work surface.

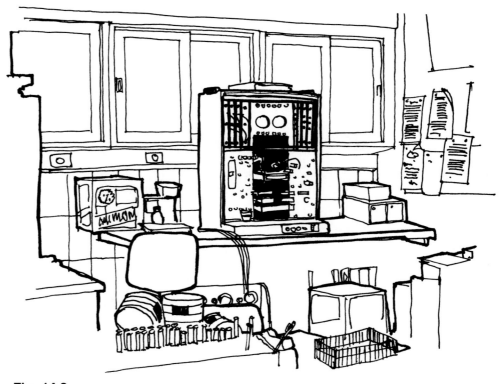

Fig. 14.2
Do not locate the blood analyzer on a fixed counter top. Placing this instrument on a moveable table allows rear access for servicing.

Evaluation of Casework Systems

> **66** *. . . The user is cautioned that although there can be considerable flexibility within a modular system, the system can become rigid outside the module.* **99**

There are a number of ways one can evaluate various casework systems. The easiest and most economical way is to contact a laboratory similar to your own where a flexible casework system has been installed recently, and ask about the performance of the system. Many times it is better to actually visit various installations and question the user firsthand. If you are planning a large laboratory, you may wish to install 10 ft or 12 ft of one or two systems and have a number of employees actually use and evaluate each system. By following one of these evaluation methods, you can form your own conclusions without the laboratory consultant, designer, or architect trying to influence your decision. It is not recommended that you conduct these evaluations with the manufacturer's representative present or at your local casework distributor's showroom. The truest opinion is given by your colleague, the daily user, who has had a firsthand opportunity to evaluate the system.

138

Auxiliary Systems

There are many areas of the laboratory that do not use casework, such as the reception and waiting area, administrative and clerical area, library, conference room, classroom, or lounge. A number of the casework manufacturers have compatible furniture systems that interface with the laboratory casework, and are even interchangeable with each other. In addition, some manufacturers have moveable office partitions or dividers that can be used in all of these areas. This allows additional flexibility because you can use the same components for office areas as well as the section supervisors' cubicles, quality control, and standard and teaching areas.

However, the user is cautioned that although there can be considerable flexibility within a modular system, the system can become rigid outside the module, i.e., the most flexible systems do not interface with other similar laboratory systems. Therefore, when a particular system is selected, one becomes tied to that particular manufacturer. Time should be taken to evaluate the type of system contemplated.

Finishes

The materials used in casework construction today are the traditional woods and metals and some of the newer materials like monolithic flakeboard, high-pressure plastic laminate, extruded vinyls, and space age injection-molded thermoplastic which is fire rated as self-extinguishing.

Brushed chrome or cast aluminum drawer pulls and hinges usually are used with heavy-duty drawer glides for institutional use. Some thermoplastic systems have integral pulls molded into the individual drawers, storage modules, or cabinets. In addition, some of the plastics have integral color throughout the material, so if the product is scratched, it will not discolor the surface. Some plastic systems have an applied finish coat, that when scratched, will reveal the natural-colored undersurface which is unsightly, especially when the stronger or darker surface colors are used.

Laboratory work surfaces or tops have always been a mystery to the user. Which material is the best? Which one does not scratch, stain, fade, burn, warp, crack, split, or delaminate? We have all asked these questions; unfortunately, there is no one material that can meet all ideal selection criteria. Therefore, it is important to know which materials are available and what the best applications are for specific work areas. Recently, a new counter-top material has been developed which is a homogenous mineral-filled acrylic polymer. It is solid and nonporous with a light color and pattern throughout. It is extremely durable and resistant to stains, odors, and damage. Only simple, routine maintenance is required to keep it clean, but abrasive cleaners and pads are recommended to remove stubborn stains and cigarette burns. Its fire performance is viewed as good with low flame spread, fuel contribution, and smoke development. Its one disadvantage is that unless it is of a proper thickness and has sufficient backup material, it has a tendency to break when excessive weight is applied. Table 14.1 addresses the major work surface materials available in today's market, what they are made of, how they hold up, and their recommended uses.

Design Configurations

One should consider unique and special designs using standard components where necessary. The most common designs are alphabet layouts using some of the following letters.

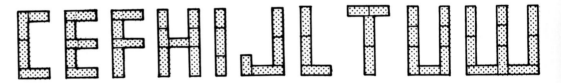

Some of the more unique or unusual designs have addressed various functional shapes:

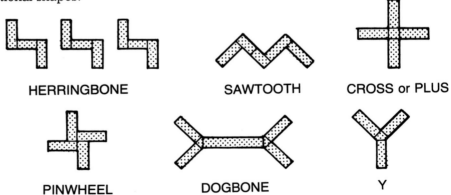

HERRINGBONE   SAWTOOTH   CROSS or PLUS

PINWHEEL   DOGBONE   Y

There also have been various modifications to work surface shape. A semicircular cut for double-headed microscope tables is the most common.

140

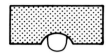

HISTOLOGY CUTTING STATION
or GENERAL WORK STATION
WITH CUTOUT

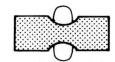

DOUBLE HEADED
SCOPE TABLE

There have been circles, squares, hexagons, and triangles:

EQUIPMENT
ISLAND WITH
KEYWAY

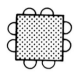

DIFFERENTIAL
TABLE

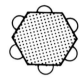

MICROBIOLOGY

MICROBIOLOGY

All of these configurations are interesting, but in most cases, not necessary. Often these designs have not been successful because they were not completely thought out, or just a whim of the designer who thought they would make an ideal work station. Most of these designs are custom built and therefore not compatible with modular systems. They may be extremely expensive to construct. Therefore, it is recommended that they be considered with care (Figs. 14.3-5).

Casework Cost

The reasons for selecting one casework system over another are many, but the final decision becomes one of cost/benefit. An effort must be made to determine the difference in the cost of the various systems through the competitive bid process. The buyer usually pays a premium of 15 percent to 20 percent more for the flexible systems.

Tax Incentives

There are three additional benefits to be gained, under current tax law, with some of the moveable systems. First, there is a 10 percent investment tax credit which is a direct reduction of federal income tax liability. Second, moveable systems can be depreciated over a five-year life compared to a 15-year life for fixed systems. The advantage here is a reduction of taxable income and tax liability and an increase in cash flow. Third, the moveable portion of the system is classified as personal property for state and local property taxes. The advantages of moveable over fixed systems are twofold as they relate to property taxes.

141

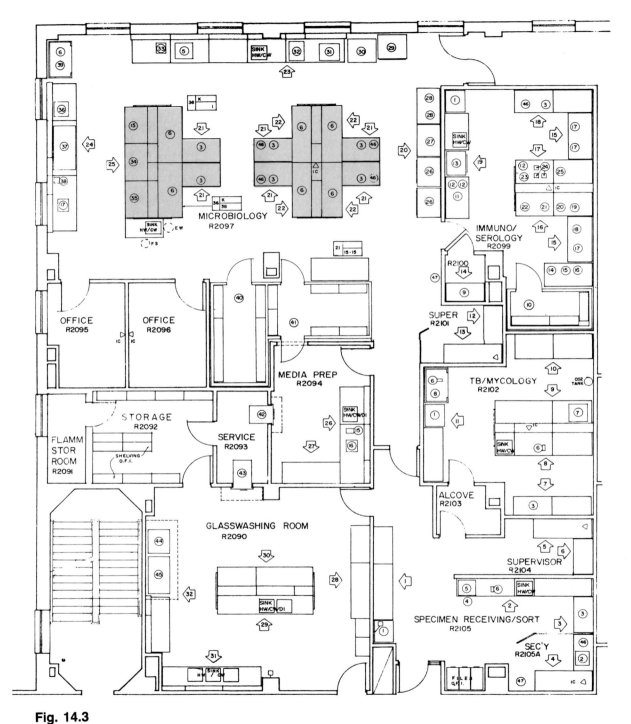

Fig. 14.3

The cross and T modules are ideal in the microbiology and blood bank areas of the laboratory.

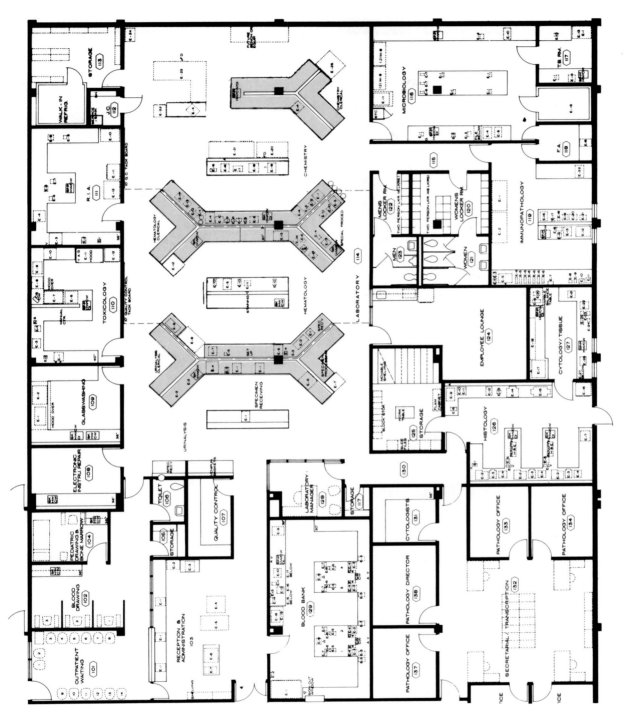

Fig. 14.4 The "dog-bone" and "Y" plans provide discrete work areas at each bench module.

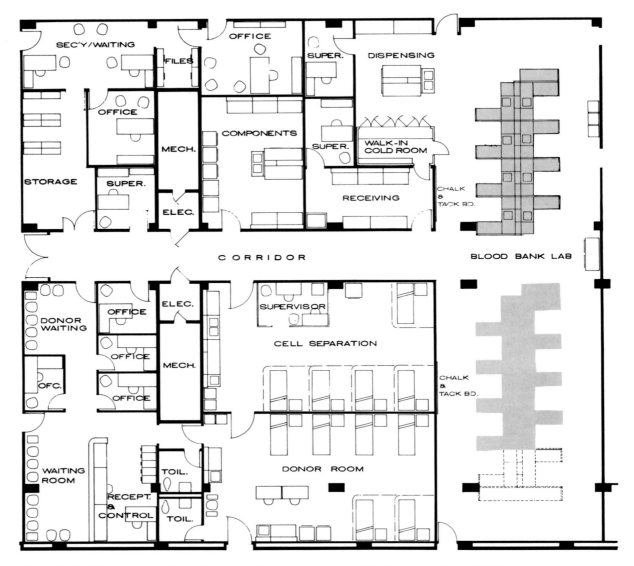

Fig. 14.5 A herringbone plan offers separate work modules within the open plan concept.

1. Moveable systems fall into the same category as furniture and fixtures. As time goes by they depreciate, thus falling into a lower tax category and, therefore, property taxes are lower.

2. Fixed systems are classified as real property and taxed at an

increasing rate. Real property in most instances is taxed at the state equalized value, which can vary from 25 percent to 100 percent of fair market value.

Before rejecting the flexible system based on cost alone it is important to review the alternatives. If one compares the flexible casework system to moveable partitions and office landscape partition systems, there is considerable data available describing the advantages of flexibility. It is estimated that after one or two major modifications the flexible system pays for itself.

It is reasonable to assume that many major changes within the laboratory occur during the initial occupancy period. Some of the reasons for this are:

1. Failure to communicate with the user during the planning process.

2. Misunderstanding of the planning documents.

3. Failure to properly demonstrate the use of the system to the user.

4. Changes of equipment programmed and not actually purchased.

5. Changes in the method of performing a procedure.

6. Changes in key personnel interviewed during the planning process.

7. Time frame from original program and planning phase to the actual occupancy and use, which can be two to three years or longer.

As was stated previously, traditional fixed casework allows for no errors or unforeseen changes. This usually means that you are forced to use the new laboratory as constructed even if the reasons described impact adversely on the daily operation.

Utilities

When laying out your laboratory, thought should be given to the type and location of the basic utilities that are required. The need for the following services must be considered:

Electrical (see NFPA 76-B: Essential Electrical Systems for Health Care Facilities)

1. *General circuits*—General circuits and receptacles should be provided throughout the laboratory. It is recommended that duplex receptacles be provided approximately 2 ft on center at the laboratory work surface in order to plug in the various pieces of equipment. It is ideal if there is one dedicated circuit per bench module which allows the user to identify an overload or defective equipment much easier and quicker. Other receptacles should be located at about 8 ft on center in offices, conference rooms, waiting rooms, lounges, etc. It is wise to provide receptacles in storage areas because there are occasions when pieces of equipment are parked and charged or set up as temporary backup modules. There should also be enough receptacles along corridors and laboratory walls for use by the housekeeping and maintenance section. It is not recommended that they plug into the electrical outlets located at the workbenches.

2. *Heavy duty or motor load circuit*—Heavy duty or motor load circuits should be separate and the receptacle or receptacle cover plate can be color coded or engraved to identify separate dedicated circuits or 220 V circuits. Usually black, brown or ivory-colored circuits are used for general (110 V) circuits and equipment and heavy duty circuits have either white and/or three-prong or twist-lock receptacles and plugs.

3. *Emergency circuit (lighting and power)*—Emergency circuits should be provided to at least one duplex receptacle at each laboratory workbench. These receptacles are colored red and have a matching cover plate. The person in charge of the laboratory should establish which equipment should be placed on the emergency circuits and should think in terms of a prolonged power outage of two to three days, rather than one or two hours. It is important that only enough equipment necessary be selected to stay operational and be able to meet all test requests. Obviously, the blood bank refrigerators should be on the emergency circuit as well as reagent and media refrigerators, selected incubators, microscopes, washing equipment, clerical equipment, and some of the necessary automated laboratory equipment. Do not take the position that all electrical services to the laboratory should be on the emergency generators. This can be extremely expensive and totally unnecessary. The electrical engineer normally will provide only the required number of emergency

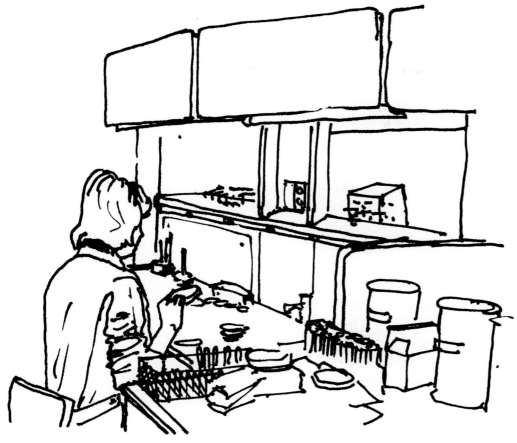

Fig. 14.6

Gas, air, electrical services, and cup sinks should be mounted on top of the utility chase in order to allow free movement of the work surface.

outlets and lighting. It is up to laboratory management to tell the laboratory consultant or the architect which additional emergency circuits must be provided (Fig. 14.6).

4. *Uninterrupted power services (UPS)*—With the large number of sophisticated electronic equipment located in today's laboratories, users are becoming increasingly aware of problems with electrical power. Minicomputers, data terminals, and electronic analyzers, etc., commonly fall victim to their own complexities. This usually occurs because electrical power can disrupt sensitive circuitry causing memory loss, malfunction, and component failure that leads to frequent service. This "dirty power" comes from transient disturbances, unstable voltage, dips and surges, noise, brownouts, and blackouts.

These conditions are overcome by using line noise suppressors, voltage stabilizers, or power conditioners. Line suppressors protect your equipment against electrical noise which occurs between the current-carrying conductors and ground, and as transverse-mode noise, which occurs between the two current-carrying conductors. Voltage stabilizers monitor line voltage and respond to fluctuations in less than one cycle of operating frequency. Power conditioners combine noise attenuation and excellent voltage regulation in one convenient system.

5. *Monitoring systems (alarms, temperature, humidity)*—Monitoring systems are not only a requirement but a necessity in today's contemporary laboratory. You are required to have an alarm connected to your blood bank refrigerators with preset temperature settings which sound an alarm when exceeded. These alarms should be located in an area (such as the hospital switchboard), which is staffed on a 24-hour basis. The maintenance section dispatch office, hospital security office, or specimen receiving desk located in the laboratory are suitable locations if staffed on a 24-hour basis. Temperature alarms also are necessary on cold rooms and walk-in incubators. Where raised floors are used, a humidity alarm and smoke detector should be installed in case of a water leak or possible fire.

6. *Communications (telephone, intercom, telewriters, paging, music, teleconferencing)*—One area that usually is neglected in overall laboratory planning is a communications network consisting of telephones, intercom, departmental paging, music, and telewriters. During the design development phase laboratory managers or chief technologists should coordinate with the architect the location of each telephone/intercom instrument and the master and submaster units. A single instrument for the telephone and intercom should be considered, rather than having two separate units which take up valuable counter or desk space. Often it is desirable to have departmental paging as part of the telephone system. This allows one to locate key personnel when necessary without having to physically search throughout the entire laboratory in order to find someone.

Background music has been used in some laboratories with limited success. It does offer a certain degree of "white sound" to help offset talking, motor noises, centrifuges, typing, and other objectionable noises. The main objection to piped in music is the limited variety and continued disagreement among employees as to what type of music to listen to. Some laboratories are presently equipping one of their conference rooms with teleconferencing capability and show inservice or continuing education programs that have become available nationwide.

7. *Word processing*—Word processors have become standard transcription equipment in laboratories, either as part of the computer system, or as a separate system. Central dictating from the gross dissecting stations, microscope reading rooms, morgue/autopsy rooms, and office areas can all be tied into the central transcription area where all reports and correspondence can be generated, distributed, and filed. Access to electrical wire-trays helps expedite installation and expansion of these systems.

Mechanical (Heating, ventilating, and air-conditioning HV/AC)
(See NFPA 56-C Laboratories in Health Related Institutions)

1. *Supply ducts*—Supply ducts are required to bring necessary fresh air into the laboratory, offices, classrooms, lounges, waiting rooms, etc. The number of air supplies is established by codes which are reviewed and revised periodically. Therefore, no effort is made to list the required air changes for various areas of the laboratory but only to alert the laboratory personnel, architect, and mechanical engineers that the air supply requirements be in compliance with all applicable codes.

2. *Return ducts*—Return or exhaust ducts also are required to remove the used air from the laboratory and the number of air exchanges should be in compliance with all applicable codes. Depending on the design of the air supply and exhaust system, it usually becomes necessary to extend duct work through corridor walls and smoke partitions, which requires the installation of smoke and fire dampers.

3. *Hood exhausts (canopy, back-draft, bonnet, chemistry, biological, laminar flow)*—Hood exhaust in laboratories is extremely important for the safety and well-being of the patients and employees in the hospital laboratory. There are numerous types of hood exhaust systems used in the laboratory which include the following:

   Canopy: This type is used over a large special chemistry workbench for exhausting odors and toxic fumes, over autoclave or sterilizer doors to capture odors and humidity, and over glass washing equipment to exhaust heat and humidity. The main disadvantage with the canopy hood is that a large amount of air is required to provide an effective exhaust velocity. There also is the danger of the operator breathing toxic materials because they may be drawn past his or her face.

Conventional hood: An enclosure in which noxious, toxic, and other harmful materials can safely be handled. The hood consists of an overall enclosure with an adjustable safety glass sash and an exhaust blower-motor at the end of the system in order to maintain a negative pressure. The exhaust ducts and blowers are separate from all other systems in the laboratory or building proper. The exhaust ducts usually are located on the roof away from fresh air intake grilles.

Back-draft: These hoods are located at the back face of the bench, usually where activities such as dissecting, cover slipping, and special staining are performed. The hood works on the same principle as the canopy hood, i.e., using large quantities of air, but in this case not allowing the fumes, odors, or toxic materials to exhaust past the user's face.

Bonnet: These hoods are located at the bench and function similarly to the canopy hood. They are used to exhaust heat from a flame photometer or other heat-generating equipment.

Radiological: These hoods are used for radioactive materials and are self-contained with integral bottoms and sides for easy decontamination. A proper base and support should be provided in the event lead shielding or leaded containers are used for storage. HEPA (High Efficiency Particulate Air, 99.97 percent efficiency) filters are used for removing harmful material from the system before it is exhausted into the atmosphere.

Biological: These hoods usually have a glove box so the operator can work within the closed chamber. They also have disposable filters which are collected in proper disposal bags and autoclaved before final disposal.

Laminar flow: This type of hood is not recommended for work with infectious materials, but rather for the preparation of sterile media, the assembly of sterile components, or examination of sterile equipment and material. Working with live agents in these hoods is not recommended. The operation of this type of hood is similar to the laminar flow hood with HEPA filters, but only protects the product or specimen from airborne contamination. It does not protect the operator.

Perchloric acid fume hood: Because of the potential explosion hazard of perchloric acid, this hood must be constructed of relatively inert materials similar to type 316 stainless steel, Alberene stone (grade 25) or ceramic-coated material. There should also be a wash-down feature incorporated because the entire hood and duct system must be completely rinsed after each use to prevent the accumulation of explosive residue. Monitoring systems should be included to assure 150 fpm open-face velocity when in operation and that the wash-down feature is activated.

4. *Extinguishing systems*—Appropriate fire extinguishing systems should be installed in canopy hoods and conventional hoods where required by code. Fire extinguishers should be provided throughout the laboratory in conjunction with required exit signs of the size, color, and style dictated by code. In computer rooms, consideration should be given to using HALON 1301 gas for extinguishing possible fires, because this chemical does not harm electrical circuits, transistors, etc. Caution should be used when working with HALON 1301 gas because when activated into an area, it displaces all available oxygen, thus extinguishing the fire. Obviously, it CAN BE HARMFUL TO HUMANS.

Plumbing (See NFPA 56-C)

1. *Natural water*—All water piped into the laboratory should be potable in quality. Unfortunately, tap water received in the laboratory is not pure enough for laboratory use. Most tap water contains calcium and magnesium bicarbonate (hardness) as well as sodium chloride (salt). Additional foreign matter includes organics, simpler ion, and nonionic compounds as well as biologic waste material and dissolved gases such as oxygen, nitrogen, and carbon dioxide. Finally, microorganisms (bacteria, fungi, viruses, protozoa, and algae) and suspended material ranging from sand to colloidal suspensions also can be found. Various treatment methods are available for the removal of most of these objectional substances and they must be used in order to produce acceptable laboratory grade water.

2. *Water treatment*—As just described, natural water is not necessarily pure. Basically, there are five methods available for producing laboratory quality water. These treatment methods are as follows:

   Filtration: Filtration of suspended material is a major step to removing unwanted material from the final-use water. This can be accomplished by the use of various types of filters. Depth type, disposable fibrous material or loose materials such as sand, anthracite, or mixed media of special characteristics are often used as filters. Membrane filters also are used and are made of cellulose acetate, polyamide, or polysulphone materials. These units must be replaced regularly because bacteria can grow through the filter element. Some types also can be cleaned and autoclaved for refuse.

Distillation: The oldest and most common method used to purify water. A still is used to vaporize the water and cooling coils to condense the vapor. The impurities are left in the heating chamber. This is the simplest method of purifying water but it does have a few disadvantages: (1) operational inefficiency, (2) extremely high maintenance cost, and (3) limited removal of volatile materials.

Deionization: This process removes ionic species by passing water through a column of ion-exchange resin beads. The degree of purification depends on the total surface area of the resin beads and the ion exchange resin in the column. However, deionized water may still contain nonionic impurities such as organics and particulate matter.

Carbon adsorption: In this method activated charcoal filters are used which, because of the large surface area of the charcoal, have the ability to absorb large amounts of organic matter. Granulated, activated charcoal filters can be used in conjunction with the deionized and reverse osmosis methods to produce top quality water. The main objection to using the system by itself is that it is difficult to avoid biological contamination.

Reverse osmosis: A reverse osmosis system uses a semipermeable membrane which removes soluble and suspended impurities. Most organics and large nonionized inorganics, bacteria, viruses, and pyrogens are removed by ultrafiltration. This method is simple and economical but it does require pretreatment of the feed water to optimize membrane life and it has a poor rejection of dissolved gases.

There are three levels of water produced by any one or a combination of the various methods just described. Their recommended uses are as follows:

Type III: For general purpose glassware cleaning and unrefined test procedures. This is comparable to CAP TYPE III, ASTM TYPE IV, or NCCLS TYPE II and can be produced by distillation, deionization, or in some localities, by reverse osmosis.

Type II: Final rinsing of glassware and more sensitive procedures usually require this caliber of water. The quality of water is produced by deionization with mixed bead resin or by double distillation. This is equal to CAP TYPE II, ASTM TYPE II or III, or NCCLS TYPE II.

Type I: For critical test procedures such as spectrometry, electrophoresis, chromatography, and fluorometric procedures, enzyme studies, and the preparation of butter solutions. This type of water can be obtained only by recirculation through nuclear grade deionization resin and charcoal and submicron filtration. The use of reverse osmosis-treated water for final processing reduces costs significantly and helps produce high purity water. This water is comparable to CAP TYPE I, ASTM TYPE I, or NCCLS TYPE I.

Once the quality of water you desire is produced, there are some remaining problems such as storage and distribution. It is recommended that only small quantities be stored in proper vessels, preferably glass or glass-lined containers. If you pipe the water throughout the laboratory a loop system is recommended as opposed to a single-line, dead-end system. In a loop system, all the water is in motion when it is discharged at any point in the loop. In a single-line, dead-end system, the end of the line may become contaminated because of inactivity. Refer to the College of American Pathologist *Reagent Water Specifications* manual for further information regarding laboratory water systems.

3. *Sinks*—Sinks should be located only where needed and in sizes, depth, and configuration required. Traditionally, sinks have been located at the end of or aisle side of a typical workbench. The necessity for water has become more selective and the use of sinks has turned from a water source to a work station for staining, glass washing, soaking, rinsing, or just a place to water aspirate or to pour off some liquid substance. Sinks are available in various sizes but they usually fit into a 2-ft-deep counter top 24 in or 48 in wide. Therefore, locate sinks where needed, and do not sacrifice valuable work surface for a sink used occasionally.

The most common materials used for sinks are resin or stainless steel, type 316. They can be attached to a plastic laminate work surface or be an integral part of a resin top. Aerators are recommended to avoid splashing, and a serrated hose end connection should be used if a length of tubing is to be attached. Usually sink sizes are 15 in wide × 18 in long × 10 in deep. These may be used as single, double, or multiple compartments depending on the need. If you wish to pour off or drain a piece of equipment, a standard cup sink (4-in × 7-in oval) can be used or the larger 6-in × 14-in rectangular cup sink may be used.

When using sinks for acid waste the architect should be informed because the plumbing engineers must specify the proper acid waste piping and a dilution basin. Consideration should be given to using acid waste piping throughout the laboratory in case the originally programmed use of a sink changes. This may be more costly but allows maximum flexibility.

4. *Standpipes and floor sinks*—The use of standpipes and floor sinks for draining blood analyzers and chemical analyzers allows drainage directly into the waste system without cluttering work surfaces and counter space. A trap primer should be installed which allows water to flow through the trap for a limited time after the equipment is turned off in order to flush any residue or remaining chemicals that may cause an obstruction or undesirable odors.

5. *Safety shower and eye wash*—These devices are required by CAP and OSHA standards and should be located throughout the laboratory in critical areas. Floor drains are not recommended under the flood shower but some states or municipalities do require them. Where drains are required they should be filled with water at least once a week to prevent the water seal from evaporating. Refer to the CAP Safety Manual, Safety Guide for Health Care Institutions AHA and National Safety Council, or OSHA regulations for laboratories.

   Drinking fountains or electric water coolers should be provided in the patient waiting areas and in various locations throughout the laboratory for the employees.

Work Space and Design Options

In planning the laboratory there are many factors that may impact on the final design. The design constraints are not always physical, financial, space availability, relationships, personnel, equipment, or communications. Within the designated design, specific functions must occur in order for these activities to interact smoothly with other areas in the laboratory. The design must address each specific task. Therefore, some basic work modules may be developed that can be used in each designated area. A work module is the space necessary for one or more persons to perform a specific task with the appropriate work surfaces, cabinetry, utilities, equipment, communications, and supplies. Some basic work modules are found in the various sections of the laboratory which may be for manual or automated procedures (Fig. 14.7). Clerical modules may be developed for such areas as specimen receiving, transcribing, and supervision. Other technical areas may be developed such as blood-drawing stations. The following lists represent some basic work modules that are typically found in a laboratory environment.

- *Differential*
- *Staining*
- *Special staining*
- *Gross dissecting*
- *Histology cutting*
- *Automated modules*

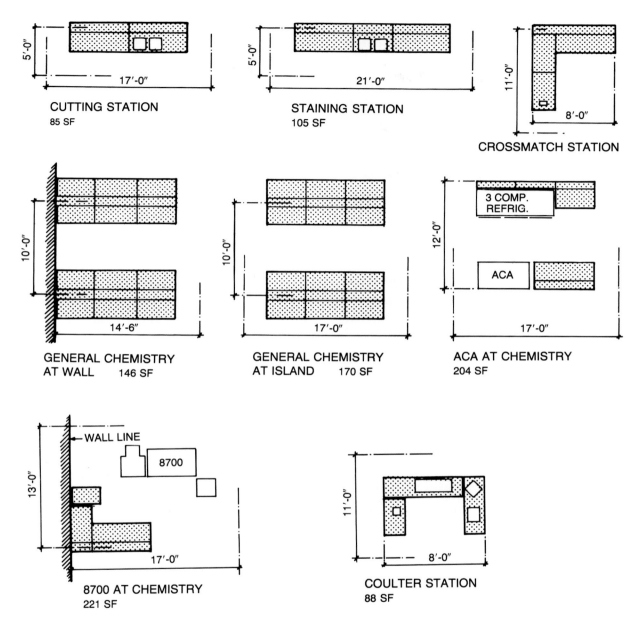

Fig. 14.7 Example of work stations.

155

Instruments and Equipment

Needless to say, the instruments and equipment in the laboratory have a considerable impact on the ultimate design. Laboratory equipment usually falls into three categories: (a) instruments, (b) equipment, and (c) nontechnical support equipment with each category requiring specific design considerations. Some examples of each category are listed in Table 14.2.

Ergonomics, Interiors and You

Today, the science of ergonomics is influencing the design of the building envelope as well as individual work spaces, furniture, lighting, and colors. Ergonomics, also known as biotechnology or human performance engineering, has been defined as "the aspect of technology concerned with the application of biological and engineering data to problems relating to man and the machine." In the June 1981 issue of *Administrative Management*, a leading authority of office design said, "A proper application of ergonomics and environmental treatment to the design of the work place will actually improve working conditions, while contributing to worker comfort and return on investment."

> **66** *. . . A work module is the space necessary for one or more persons to perform a specific task with the appropriate work surfaces, cabinetry, utilities, equipment, supplies, and communications.* **99**

Table 14.2

Laboratory Instruments and Equipment

INSTRUMENTS	EQUIPMENT	SUPPORT EQUIPMENT
Microscope	Refrigerators	Chairs
Spectrophotometer	Freezers	Desks
Flame photometer	Centrifuge	Stools
PH Meter/Blood gases	Incubators/drying ovens	File cabinets
Automated analyzer	Microtome	Fire cabinets
Coagulyzer	Hoods	Metal shelving
Fibrometer	Waterbath	CRT
Blood cell counter	Timers	Typewriters
Gas chromatograph	Hot plates	Acid storing cabinet
Gamma counter	Autoclaves	Waste receptacles

Laboratory furniture manufacturers have developed flexible or changeable work modules which begin to address the personal and public spatial experience on the basis of individual behavior in varying situations. The need to adjust work counters, shelves, and task lighting is only a small part of an efficient, productive, and nonfatiguing work environment. Depth of counters and shelves plays an equally important part in creating the ideal work space but the obvious basics like chairs, reaching for a phone or reference material, and color and texture of work surfaces all contribute to a safe and productive work place.

Chair and stool selection is extremely important because a number of people may use the same seating for prolonged periods. The seating selected must be able to accommodate a 5-ft, 100-lb woman to a 6-ft man weighing 200 lb. This is accomplished by selecting easily adjusted seating with hydraulic cylinders which can change height by simply depressing a small lever located under the seat. More importantly, the person using the seat must take the time to make the necessary adjustments and must be encouraged by their supervisor to do so. Adjustment of the back-rest tension further adds to the comfort of the user (Fig. 14.8).

It is recommended that the ceiling lighting be installed diagonally or perpendicular to the workbench. This distributes a uniform light pattern and

Fig. 14.8

The use of flexible laboratory furniture with adjustable work surfaces allows the operator to work at a comfortable and nonfatiguing height. Chairs of the proper height and stools with adjustable back rests also are recommended.

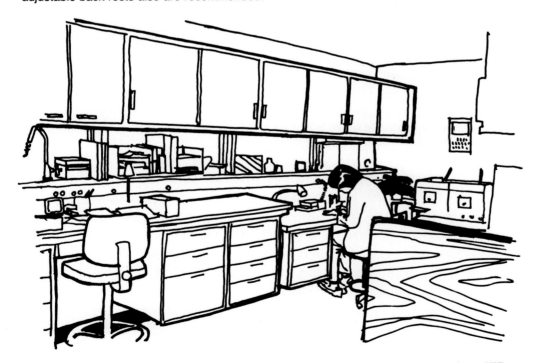

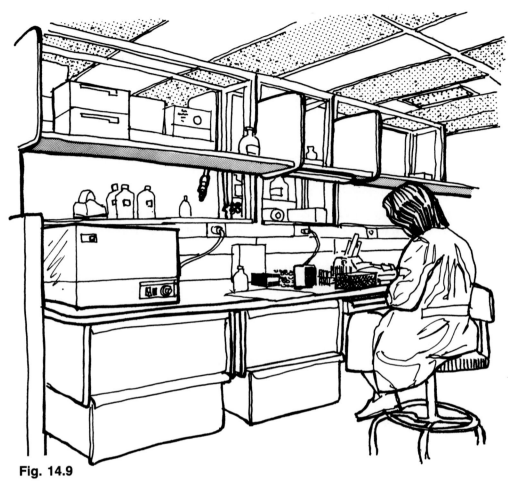

Fig. 14.9

The ceiling lighting is designed perpendicular to the work surface in order to avoid working in your own shadow. Task light is located under the overhead cabinet and provides additional light where needed.

avoids working in your own shadow. Task lighting (under cabinet lights) can augment the overhead light and provide a specific light source at the work surface (Fig. 14.9).

Laboratory furniture manufacturers now offer a rainbow of accent colors which, when used with an off-white or neutral overall color, enhances the work environment. One should strive for a human comfort factor and try to warm up the area with some wood tones, draperies, plants, and a few pictures.

For the past 30 to 40 years architects and mechanical engineers have strived to create a total building environment by designing buildings without op-

158

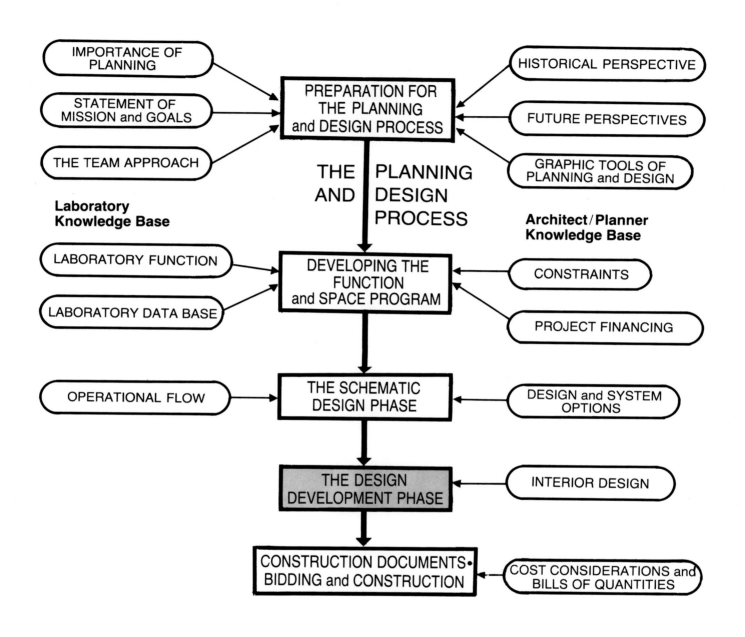

IMPORTANCE OF PLANNING

STATEMENT OF MISSION and GOALS

THE TEAM APPROACH

PREPARATION FOR THE PLANNING and DESIGN PROCESS

HISTORICAL PERSPECTIVE

FUTURE PERSPECTIVES

GRAPHIC TOOLS OF PLANNING and DESIGN

THE PLANNING AND DESIGN PROCESS

Laboratory Knowledge Base

Architect/Planner Knowledge Base

LABORATORY FUNCTION

LABORATORY DATA BASE

DEVELOPING THE FUNCTION and SPACE PROGRAM

CONSTRAINTS

PROJECT FINANCING

OPERATIONAL FLOW

THE SCHEMATIC DESIGN PHASE

DESIGN and SYSTEM OPTIONS

THE DESIGN DEVELOPMENT PHASE

INTERIOR DESIGN

CONSTRUCTION DOCUMENTS• BIDDING and CONSTRUCTION

COST CONSIDERATIONS and BILLS OF QUANTITIES

Part IV
THE DESIGN DEVELOPMENT PHASE

DESIGN DEVELOPMENT 15

The objective of the design development phase is for the architect and engineers to resolve all issues affecting both the design and detailed development of the building. At the end of the design development phase, all decisions should be made which affect the development of the construction documents and actual initiation of construction. The design development phase is a period in which many details are determined. It is not a continuation of the schematic design phase; the decisions which were made during this phase are still firm. The design development documents simply explore and resolve the detailed issues required to translate the schematic documents into construction drawings. At this point, the laboratory representatives continue to be involved in the development of the documents. Detailed decisions on types of fixtures, specific placement of items, and development of casework are made during this phase. In conjunction with the architect's development of documents, the equipment planning effort is in full force and has provided the design team, including the architect and engineers, with detailed specifications for each major piece of fixed and moveable equipment.

At this stage, single-line drawings become more specific. For instance, rather than being a single stroke of a pen, a wall section may now be represented as one layer of ⅝-in gypsum board on each side of a metal stud, etc. This level of detail is pursued by all the design disciplines. The structural engineer is making final calculations on loads and structural requirements. Specific components of the structural system are being determined and the final dimensions are being coordinated with the architectural and engineering documents. Likewise, the mechanical, plumbing, and electrical engineers are further refining their systems. As these issues are resolved and developed, there is coordination between all the design disciplines.

The involvement of the laboratory representatives continues at this point to ensure that their understanding of the design is complete. They also have input in making decisions on specific details.

In order to complete the design of casework and laboratory furniture, it is necessary to make choices between all the various systems available. Once again, coordination with all the other activities in the design process is vital even in the selection of casework. The laboratory must accommodate space for people, equipment, and fixed and moveable furniture. Each piece of casework should be selected and designed with the specific function in mind. The height should be evaluated in terms of the desired position in which a person works. Will the technician be standing or sitting? If there is a combination of both, then the solution may be in the type of stool on which the technician sits rather than the height of the casework. Location and types of utilities to the casework must be considered.

It is unwise to simply provide an overall blanket of utilities and services to all areas of the laboratory. This creates unnecessary costs and inhibits flexibility in rearranging the layout in the future. It is helpful to develop utilities along the lines of wet and dry areas. Portions of casework or work stations may be designated as wet areas or for dry procedures and instrumentation. Hopefully, it is possible to provide areas which may be totally moveable. Thoughtful placement of wet sink areas and permanent plumbing items provides easy access by technicians.

Another area which involves choices is in the interior design of the environment. The interior design may be done by the architect or another specialized person. The selection of materials must meet requirements for performance before those of esthetic appeal. Laboratory workbenches are traditionally an item for which material selection has been difficult and often unsatisfactory. Requirements for safety and code compliance also limit the materials available and how they are used. Building and life safety codes for fireproofing, smoke generation, and flame spread characteristics of materials are specified in the laboratory. The maintenance and durability of materials must be considered. Qualities such as acoustics, light, brightness, variety, and mood also affect the interior design. While it may not be necessary to finalize the specific material and color selections at this time, it is necessary to establish the overall criteria and types of materials to be used so that coordination with the wall systems, details, and the transition of materials can be resolved.

The development of these detailed decisions should involve the analysis

> *" . . . Coordination with all the other activities in the design process is vital . . ."*

and evaluation of several options. The project team should continue to be involved as a group in making these selections. At this level of development, it is possible to evaluate performance criteria specifically, as well as relative cost of a number of different systems.

The site plan is also developed at this stage. Any site grading and utility development is explored and all potential conflicts removed. Soil and other subsurface testing should be provided if not already complete.

The vertical component of the building now is considered in the design process. Detailed decisions on the materials for the outside walls, windows and door openings, roofing materials, and other support systems influence the performance and physical appearance of the building. The architect is dealing with issues involving the energy efficiency of the building through control of light and heat, etc.

The site design should be considered in detail. Performance for function and flow of the site may be analyzed in much the same manner as the function and flow of the laboratory work station. Employees need to park or otherwise be accommodated as they arrive for work. Material suppliers and trash removal service requires access to the site and circulation to specific points of the building. The orientation of the building and identification of it may be important for both ease of access to persons coming to the area and perhaps as a means of marketing the services available in the laboratory. It is important that this be considered at this stage so that the scope of work to be anticipated and the level to which costs are incurred can be factored into the project budget.

At the completion of the design development phase, a third review and formal approval process occurs. At this time, it may be necessary to submit the plans for review and approval by government agencies. The project team must make a thorough review of decisions made up to this point and compare these with the assumptions and requirements specified in the previous stages. An updated cost estimate may be developed from the design development documents, and the most accurate evaluation of the project cost presented at this time. After all this information is available, a specific decision is made to proceed into the contract documents.

Contract Documents

The contract documents or working drawings and specifications are the final documents on which the architect and design engineers specifically illustrate the configuration of the building. It is important that these documents be as comprehensive and intelligible as possible to all the team members. They typically include drawings and written specifications for all aspects of the building construction.

Specifications are a part of the contract documents, including the working drawings, any addenda, and the agreements between the owner and the contractor. The specifications consist of written requirements for materials, equipment, construction systems, standards, and workmanship. See the bibliography for recommended references on the subject.

The CSI Construction Index

Many hospitals' construction projects are bid or negotiated using the Construction Specifications Institute (CSI) classification of work according to 16 divisions. These divisions recognize the distinct contracting specialties and vendors that are used in a construction project. They can form a useful framework for budgeting and monitoring project costs and for preparing and monitoring project schedules, even if their use is not required for formal procedures.

A sample listing with subdivisions of the 16 major divisions used can be found in Appendix D. The 16 major divisions are listed here, with a few examples of how they might be used in a laboratory project.

DIVISION	DESCRIPTION
1	General requirements
2	Sitework
3	Concrete
4	Masonry
5	Metals
6	Wood and plastic
7	Thermal and moisture protection
8	Doors and windows
9	Finishes
10	Specialties
11	Equipment
12	Furnishings
13	Special construction
14	Conveying systems
15	Mechanical
16	Electrical

A group of items or services to be included in a laboratory project, such as a walk-in refrigerator, is assigned a five-digit number. Laboratory furniture, for example, has been assigned the number 12345. The CSI does not explicitly recognize so-called moveable equipment, but those items can be thought of as belonging to one or more specially created divisions.

At least one compendium of manufacturer's brochures and specifications is organized by the CSI 16-division system; that is, Sweets Catalog, published by McGraw Hill Information Systems in New York City. This multivolume set is used by many construction professionals and can be helpful in selecting and evaluating sources for products and services.

The laboratory representatives on the project team have limited involvement during the contract document stage. This activity is focused on providing construction information and final coordination of all the disciplines. Most of the decisions requiring input from the owner and user should have been made at this time, because it is difficult and costly to make changes after this phase.

" . . . Coordination with all the other activities in the design process is vital . . ."

More than likely, a schedule is developed for the initiation and completion of the construction activities. The project team should review this schedule and the ways that it impacts on the operation of the laboratory. If the project is an expansion or renovation, the logistics and coordination in maintaining operations while construction is underway must be analyzed by all members of the team. They should be concerned with minimizing the disruption to current operations.

When the contract documents are complete, the building is ready for construction. It is now possible to define an accurate cost for the project and in fact fix that cost, depending on the construction methodology. At this stage, government agencies may require a final review and approval cycle and the owner also must review and approve documents for construction.

INTERIOR DESIGN 16

AFTER THE LABORATORY SIZE, departmental relationships, space allocations, flow, and management have been resolved, the remaining element of major importance is the esthetic environment. For years most hospitals had dull and drab environments on the premise that an institution should have an institutional look. The argument for using all white or pea-green wall paint, and later beige, was that the hospital did not have to inventory numerous colors. It was easier to keep the light colors aseptically clean and it was easier to paint everything the same color. Fortunately, hospitals have become more humanized and colorful with some dramatic effects.

On entering a hospital, the laboratory is one of the technical areas that the patient sees first, be it the main laboratory or the admitting or outpatient laboratory. These areas should be attractive with textured wall surfaces of washable, heavy-duty vinyl fabrics or accent-painted walls with beautiful harmonizing colors. It is not recommended that wood paneling be used in this environment because, in order to meet the fire codes, the cost of paneling becomes prohibitive. Draperies should be used whenever possible to provide texture, color, and pattern as well as a degree of sound control. Do not hesitate to use drapes on walls without windows; this helps add color and sound absorption to such areas as conference rooms, offices, interior waiting rooms, lounges, and some laboratory work areas. The use of drapes has been effective in controlling sound in computer rooms and around computer equipment such as printers and labelers. Centrifuge stations can be surrounded by 60-in or 80-in-high sound-absorbing partitions, which are upholstered with colorful accents or attractive patterns.

The patient waiting areas are especially important and should include paintings, framed prints, wall hangings, landscaping, and attractive, comfortable furniture. It is important that these areas convey a feeling of welcome and confidence and help to set the patient at ease, especially since this may be their first visit to the hospital.

169

Every effort should be made to make the patient comfortable, but it is equally important to establish an attractive work environment for the laboratory personnel who occupy these spaces on a daily basis.

Attractive employee lounge areas with coffee bar, microwave oven, sink, and refrigerator to store their lunches is strongly recommended. The furniture should be well constructed, attractively designed, and most of all comfortable. Provisions should be made for employee locker facilities where personal clothing and items can be kept. Many times employees are asked to share lockers with someone but half-lockers can be purchased which occupy only a few inches more of floor space and offer each employee a private locker. This area should have a full-length mirror and some seating.

The patient and employee toilets should be located near the waiting room, locker room, or lounge, respectively. If possible, it is desirable to locate the patient toilets in such a manner that specimens can be collected and passed directly to the laboratory without having to walk through the waiting room or through a public corridor.

Carpeting used to be a status symbol and still is in some institutions. Because of the many advantages of carpeting, e.g., sound control, comfort, warmth, texture and color, it is being used more. Primary areas for carpeting are the reception and waiting rooms, offices, conference and teaching rooms, lounges and dressing or locker rooms. Presently, many institutions are using wall carpet in waiting rooms, lounges, dictation, and transcription rooms. Wall carpeting is available in various colors and textures and is applied directly to the wall surface like vinyl wall covering. It is especially effective in noisy areas such as the computer printing area, bursting, and in centrifuge alcoves. All fabrics, vinyls, paints, and carpeting materials should meet all applicable codes for flame spread, toxicity, combustibility, and be static-free when required.

Two design concepts that have not been fully explored and used in the laboratory are graphics and signage. Graphics encompasses many areas and can include murals, photomurals, sculpture walls, graphics, and super graphics. Murals are usually a scene which has been hand drawn by an artist directly on to the wall surface using acrylic resin paints. Photomurals depict landscapes, seascapes, skylines, or enlarged photos of actual people or events. Photomurals may depict the original laboratory, hospital building, or complex. They are effective in depicting historic events. Wall sculpture is a three-dimensional bas-relief of geometric design which, when properly lighted, causes some interesting shadow effects. Super graphics depict large geometric shapes or lettering which can be used in lobbies, corridors, and open walls.

Signage should accomplish the two basic functions of giving information and identification. All too often there is no signage program in an institution and this generates many different signs in varying size, color, design, and texture. It is strongly recommended that all signage be designed and executed by one person or office and that it be uniform in size, letter style, color, and method of fastening. A good sign is one located where it can be seen easily, with legible lettering in contrasting colors with the background, and with brief text so it may be read while in motion.

All of these services, i.e., interior design, furniture selection and specification, artwork, office landscaping, murals, graphics and signage, are normally not a part of the architectural contract. This means that these services are in addition to basic architectural services. Depending on the size of your architectural firm, they may be available through the architect or by separate contracts with each specific discipline. Professional fees for these services vary. They normally are quoted as a percentage (10 percent to 20 percent) of the cost of the products bought, a lump sum/fixed fee, or a multiple-plus benefits. Reimbursable costs are billed separately and include travel and living expenses, long-distance phone calls, special mail, cost of reproduction, models, renderings, and photographs.

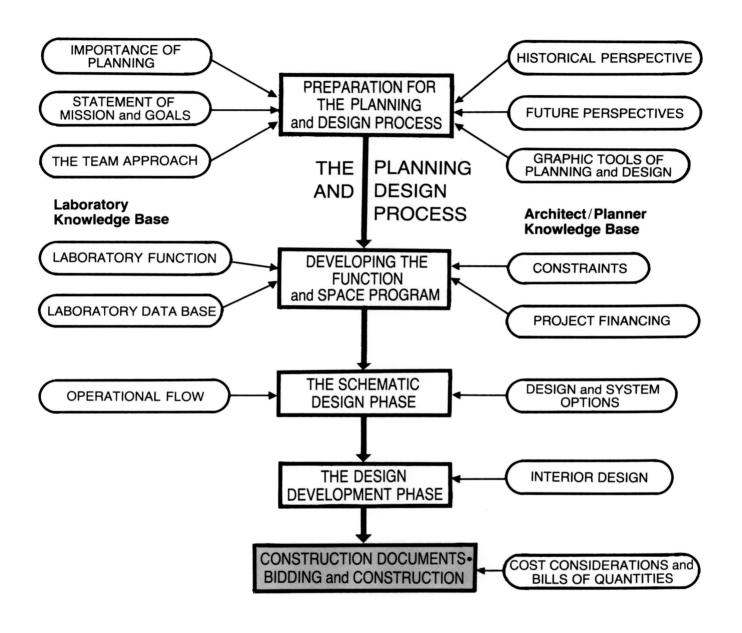

IMPORTANCE OF PLANNING

STATEMENT OF MISSION and GOALS

THE TEAM APPROACH

PREPARATION FOR THE PLANNING and DESIGN PROCESS

HISTORICAL PERSPECTIVE

FUTURE PERSPECTIVES

GRAPHIC TOOLS OF PLANNING and DESIGN

THE PLANNING AND DESIGN PROCESS

Laboratory Knowledge Base

Architect/Planner Knowledge Base

LABORATORY FUNCTION

LABORATORY DATA BASE

DEVELOPING THE FUNCTION and SPACE PROGRAM

CONSTRAINTS

PROJECT FINANCING

OPERATIONAL FLOW

THE SCHEMATIC DESIGN PHASE

DESIGN and SYSTEM OPTIONS

THE DESIGN DEVELOPMENT PHASE

INTERIOR DESIGN

CONSTRUCTION DOCUMENTS• BIDDING and CONSTRUCTION

COST CONSIDERATIONS and BILLS OF QUANTITIES

Part V
CONSTRUCTION DOCUMENTS, BIDDING, AND CONSTRUCTION

THE CONSTRUCTION PROCESS 17

PREPARATION AND CONSTRUCTION ACTIVITY BEGINS in various ways. The objective is to determine a specific cost, select a contractor, arrange for the financing, acquire the necessary permits and approvals, and set a date for initiation of the construction. There are several ways a contractor may be engaged for this project:

1. *Competitive bidding*—This involves the distribution of the contract documents to a preselected or open group of bidders. They each prepare a price estimate and bid proposal based on the construction documents. The bids are then reviewed, and based on a pre-established criteria, a bidder's proposal is selected. The qualification of the firms making the bids should be reviewed. Their ability to perform the work should be demonstrated and, in many cases, guaranteed through use of performance bonds or other measures. The bidders should be familiar with the project, site, and what is expected of them. The quality of the construction documents have the greatest affect on the accuracy and comparability of each of the bid proposals. The effort expended by the bidding firm in analyzing the documents and the cost impacts implied therein are critical to the formulation of a bid. The selection process may be based on the basis of the lowest cost bid proposal or more often, on an evaluation of the best value proposed. This would mean some evaluation of the bids cost in conjunction with the quality and performance record of the contractor making the proposal.

2. *Negotiated bid*—In private projects, competitive bidding is not mandatory. The owner may negotiate a price with one contractor. While this process does not guarantee lowest price, the owner is able to select a contractor known for high quality performance. Also, the contractor can be engaged earlier (e.g., during the design process) in order to provide expertise on cost, alternative material, and bidding assembly systems.

3. *Construction manager*—In this method, the owner engages a construction

175

manager at an early stage of the project, usually when the architect begins the schematic design. The construction manager usually is engaged on a percentage-fee basis. Construction management services are offered by affiliates of construction companies, architectural firms, or independent construction management companies. The construction manager can be useful particularly on large and complex projects. Cost-effectiveness of the construction manager on a small project may be questionable. One of the services provided by the construction manager is the monitoring of the estimated construction cost throughout the design phases. The owner gets an idea of the probable construction cost at an early stage. The construction manager also provides the architect with comparative costs of materials and building assembly systems, and may be asked by the owner to provide a guaranteed maximum price (GMP). This assures the owner that the cost of construction does not go above a certain amount. The GMP may be useful in getting financial commitments from lending institutions. Because the construction manager builds some margin into the GMP, it usually is higher than a competitive bid price.

4. *Owner as general contractor*—Many institutions have construction personnel on staff. On small to medium-size projects, the inhouse construction personnel may act as the general contractor and secure subcontractors through competitive bidding.

Once construction has begun, situations develop which may require that modifications be made to the design documents. At this time, field sketches are issued which address the specific problems as they arise. Field sketches are generally prepared and approved by the architect. It would be the architect's responsibility to ensure that the modifications proposed do not materially affect the performance outlined in the contract documents. These changes should be reviewed with the owner/user.

During the construction phase and since a certain period of time has elapsed, modifications to equipment purchase or even procedures in the laboratory may have occurred. If this is the case, it should be evaluated in terms of the proposed design being built and decisions made as to whether any changes are necessary. This is not a time to redesign the laboratory. However, it is wise to monitor the construction activity. During the final stages of construction activity, the architect and/or owner conducts an inspection and survey of the work being performed. Any deficiencies must be noted and brought to the attention of the contractor for correction. This is often referred to as the punch list. All items which are not in conformance with the contract document must be noted and brought to the contractor's attention. It is the contractor's responsibility to correct any of these situations and provide complete conformance. Also at this time, the local building inspectors make their final inspections.

Fast-Track Design and Construction

Obviously, the time spent in design and construction impact the cost of the completed project. It has become a common practice to undertake a fast-track design process in order to expedite the construction time. This is a process in which the design and the construction activity overlap. It is not an alternative to any design activity.

The basis of the fast-track process is to establish parameters for the structural grid and foundations as early as possible. Once the site, foundation, and structural package have been designed, it may be bid on and construction begun while the design and detail development continues.

This process is desirable only when it is believed that the decisions developed later in the design will not impact the decisions made at the outset concerning the structural grid. If early concensus on structural systems can be achieved, significant savings in terms of schedule and budget can be realized. Before choosing this process, local agencies which approve new plans and issue building permits must be consulted for their ability and willingness to review and approve the documents in this manner.

Post-Occupancy Review

After the new facility has been occupied and in operation for some time, it is valuable to reassemble the project team and do a post-occupancy review. This is an opportunity for the team to evaluate their process and relate the problems and successes realized. At this time, assumptions made during the initial planning phases can be reassessed and evaluated in terms of the experience of the people using the facility. Evaluating performance of materials and equipment selected is done. It may be in the best interest of the owner, architect, engineers, and contractor to examine the success of the final product. The owner and user have specific opinions on how successful the design is, and they have constructive and useful suggestions for improving the final product and perhaps even the design process for achieving this product.

COST CONSIDERATIONS AND BILLS OF QUANTITIES 18

IN ORDER TO PREPARE A BID for a construction project, it is necessary to prepare a detailed quantity survey of the labor and material resources required to complete the project. Also required is a mark-up to cover the various overheads and profit to complete the bid price.

The ability of a construction firm to win a contract therefore relies not only on the profit margin required, but its ability to purchase the specified materials at favorable rates and to organize the operational sequences in a well-ordered, methodical fashion.

The construction firm's ability to make a profit clearly relies heavily on the accuracy of the bid preparation (i.e., the quantity survey) and this in turn relies on how well the estimators and planners have interpreted the architectural/engineering drawings and specifications. This is particularly critical when it is considered that the average bid period is around four weeks and, at any given time, a construction firm must be preparing bids for six to ten projects in the anticipation of winning one contract. Several observations on this situation are important.

For a firm to carry out a detailed quantity survey of each project it bids for, and still allow time for pricing, subcontract quotations, and resource planning, the cost burden to the construction firm will be substantial. If the firm receives orders at a ratio of 1:6 or 1:10, then the burden of the unsuccessful contracts must be carried by the successful contract. Considering the time available for bid preparation and the number of bids being prepared, a risk for error must be present. Also, misinterpretation of drawings and specifications is possible. Thus, the risk of profit loss can be considerable, i.e., a risk to both the building owner and the construction firm. The building owner may accept a bid which is in effect incomplete, either too high or too low. The contractor can run the considerable risk of failing to make a reasonable profit, or sustain a substantial loss. A system of bidding which aids the contractor in preparing an accurate bid, allows the contractor to do the following: (1) use resources to study drawings and specifications in greater detail; (2) provides data which can be priced quickly; (3) allows the contractor to obtain quotations from subcontractors; and (4) provides the building owner with greater security in receiving bids.

Bills of Quantities

This document is a comprehensive list of all the items of work which the construction firm is required to cover in its bid. It also includes a list of responsibilities that the construction firm bears during the contract period (e.g., the legal contract conditions; safety, health, and welfare conditions, etc.).

The concept of Bills of Quantities is most commonly used to describe units of work "in place," that is to say, measured items of work as finished in the building, and these units include the labor and materials necessary to achieve them. Bills of Quantities, however, can be structured (sorted) in several different ways. For example:

- *By trades*
- *By work sections*
- *By elements*
- *By operational sequences*

Computer techniques can be applied to Bills of Quantities, thus providing the option of various sorting. When complete, the Bills of Quantities represent a complete description of the work shown on the architect's drawings, together with the quantity of each item of work. In order to complete the bid, the construction firm must place unit prices against each work item and the quantity multiplied by these unit rates. The total of all these extensions represents the bid price.

The Bills of Quantities is prepared by a specialist known as a quantity surveyor, who has been involved in the project with the architect/engineer over the design period, and thus is in a position to be familiar with the project as it develops. As has been stated already, the unpriced Bills of Quantities would be issued to the bidding construction firm along with the drawings and specifications.

Advantages of Bills of Quantities

These might be summarized as follows:

1. To leave a minimum of doubt as to what is covered by the bid price.

2. To ensure that all bidders calculate their bids on the same data, thereby placing them on an equal footing and reducing their bidding risks: the competition between them is therefore entirely on a financial basis and they do not have to make provision for errors in calculating their own quantities.

3. To provide a basis for financial control during the construction stages; including a basis for setting the charges for change orders.

4. To economize on the manpower required to prepare bids and on the cost involved, with anticipated project cost savings.

5. To derive the costs from Bills of Quantities which can form the basis of a valuable data bank of cost information.

6. To be used as a management tool in the preparation of the construction program.

7. To be used for ordering materials.

Bid Contracts

A frequent criticism from contractors not used to bidding on this basis is that by supplying details of unit prices they would be disclosing valuable commercial information and contributing to their own self-destruction. This should not be the case. The priced Bills of Quantities should be considered a confidential document between the building owner and the contractor. Only the professional quantity surveyor need have a copy. Bid evaluation should be only on the lump sum price, and guarantee of this should be provided to the construction firms by inviting only the successful firm to submit the complete Bills of Quantities after selection. Even when using this information for a cost data bank, confidentiality can be preserved by the method adopted for analyzing and storing the cost data.

Negotiated Contracts

Bills of Quantities are equally valuable in negotiated contracts and serve as an accurate basis for negotiating procedures. In this case, individual unit rates may be negotiated by the quantity surveyor on behalf of the building owner and, in this way, an agreed negotiated price for the building is reached.

Bills of Quantities and Performance Specifications

Since Bills of Quantities are always associated with the architect/engineer specifications and drawings, and since there is considerable flexibility possible in the method of preparing them, it is possible to closely link Bills of Quantities with performance specifications. In this case, the unit items are described relative to the performance specification, and measured quantities are provided as appropriate. The facility for the contractor to insert quantities where this would be required under the performance specification section can be provided, thus allowing the contractors the freedom to describe clearly their method of achieving the required performance standards.

Bills of Quantities and Construction Management

By using an appropriate sortation, Bills of Quantities can be of continuing value to the construction manager in planning and organizing the construction program. Sorted into operational sequences, they can become part of network planning with each sequence's associated costs forming the basis of financial control of the contract.

Bills may be sorted to provide for material orders and subcontract awards. The unit rates provide an accurate basis for preparing regular progress payment authorizations. In addition, the descriptive nature of the Bills of Quantities provides a useful "aide-memoir" of operations and materials to be provided.

Bills of Quantities as a Basis of Cost Data Bank

One of the outstanding advantages of Bills of Quantities is that they provide a unique supply of cost data which, if harnessed, can become the basis of a valuable cost information service.

Cost data of this nature can be used as a basis for setting cost limits; preparing cost plans and estimates; evaluating bids; establishing regional cost variations and, by using cost indices, determining the rate of building cost inflation.

It is important, however, that the cost information is analyzed and stored in such a way as to preserve the confidentiality of the source. This can be readily done, and construction firms may be assured of this feature.

BIBLIOGRAPHY

1. Allen RW, Karolyi IV: *Hospital Planning Handbook.* New York/London/Sydney/Toronto, John Wiley and Sons, 1976.

2. Baer DM: Designing your laboratory. *In* Stefanini M (ed): *Progress in Clinical Pathology.* New York, Grune and Stratton, 1975.

3. Bailey RW: *Human Performance Engineering—A Guide for System Designers*, Inglewood, NJ, Prentice-Hall, Inc., 1982.

4. Barker JH: *Laboratory Facilities Planning and Design*, US Department of Health, Education, and Welfare. Atlanta, Centers for Disease Control, 1982.

5. Barker JH: Total modular concept in laboratory design. *Lab Management*, September 1975, pp. 33-35.

6. Burgess JH: *Human Factors in Built Environments.* Newtonville, Mass, Environmental Design and Research Center, 1981.

7. Commission on Laboratory Accreditation: *Inspection Checklists.* Skokie, Ill, College of American Pathologists, 1983.

8. Commission on Laboratory Inspection and Accreditation: *Reagent Water Specifications.* Skokie, Ill, College of American Pathologists, 1978.

9. Elin RJ, Robertson EA, Sever G: Departmental resources and statistics of academic pathology. *Am J Clin Pathol 1981;75:662-670.*

10. Elin RJ, Robertson EA, Sever G: Workload, space, and personnel of hematology laboratories in teaching hospitals. *Am J Clin Pathol 1983;80:190-196.*

11. Elin RJ, Robertson EA, Sever G: Workload, space, and personnel of microbiology laboratories in teaching hospitals. *Am J Clin Pathol 1984;82:78-84.*

12. Everett K, Huges D: *A Guide to Laboratory Design.* London/Boston, Butterworths, 1975.

13. Haber SL: Flexibility in laboratory design as an adjunct to efficient automation. *In* Westlake GE, Bennington JT (eds): *Automation and Management in the Clinical Laboratory.* Baltimore, University Park Press, 1972.

14. Hamilton Laboratory Tops and Work Surfaces: Two Rivers, Wis, Hamilton Industries, 1976.

15. Hardy OB, Lammers LP: *Hospitals—The Planning and Design Process.* Germantown, Md, Aspen Systems Corporation, 1976.

16. Hawk WA: *Guidelines for Laboratory Safety.* Skokie, Ill, College of American Pathologists, 1984.

17. Hellmuth, Obata, and Kassabaum, Inc (Architects): Convertible laboratory furniture. Arch Record 1963;**134** (August), 169-172.

18. Koenig AS: *Laboratory Instrument Verification and Maintenance Manual*, ed 3. Skokie, Ill, College of American Pathologists, 1982.

19. Lundberg GD: *Managing the Patient-focused Laboratory.* Oradell, NJ, Medical Economics Co, 1975.

20. National Bureau of Standards, US Department of Commerce. *Safe Handling of Radioactive Materials*, NCRP Report #30.

21. *Laboratories in Health Related Institutions*, NFPA 56-C. Quincy, Mass, National Fire Protection Association, 1980.

22. *Essential Electrical System for Health Care Facilities*, NFPA 76-B. Quincy, Mass, National Fire Protection Association, 1980.

23. Newell JE: *Laboratory Management.* Boston, Little Brown and Co, 1972.

24. Public Health Service, Division of Hospital and Medical Facilities, *Planning the Laboratory for the General Hospital*, PHS Pub. No. 930-D-10, March 1963.

25. Pusch AL, et al: Planning a satellite laboratory for ambulatory patient care. *Hosp Topics* 1971;**49**:55-60.

26. Rappoport AE: *Manual for Laboratory Planning and Design.* Chicago, College of American Pathologists, 1960.

27. Ruys T: Flexibility and the concept of the basic module: flexibility in laboratory design. *Lab Management* 1970;8(pt I):22-23.

28. Ruys T: How flexible are existing laboratories? Flexibility in laboratory design. *Lab Management* 1970;8(pt V):24-28.

29. Ruys T: 37 keys to laboratory design. *Res/Dev* 1969;20:18-25.

30. Ruys T: Laboratory furniture selection. *Hospitals* 1970;44:64-66.

31. Ruys T: Projecting need for change: flexibility in laboratory design. *Lab Management* 1970;8(pt III):28-29.

32. Ruys T: The planning module: flexibility in laboratory design. *Lab Management* 1970;8(pt II):24-27.

33. Ruys T: Types of flexibility: flexibility in laboratory design. *Lab Management* 1970;8(pt IV):20-24.

34. Sydlowski W: Improve business with ergonomics. *Graphic Arts Monthly*, October 1983, pp. 118-124.

35. Thiel CT (ed): *Ergonomic Furniture: productivity by Design.* Infosystems, pp. 30-38, 1983.

36. Thomas RG: *Manual for Laboratory Planning and Design.* Skokie, Ill, College of American Pathologists, 1977.

37. Werner M, Abraham AA: Defining and defeating biohazards in the laboratory. *Med Lab Observer.* July 1981, pp. 81-97.

38. Wheeler TE: *Hospital Design and Function.* New York/San Francisco/Toronto/London, McGraw-Hill Book Co, 1964.

39. Wheeler TE: *Hospital Modernization and Expansion,* New York, McGraw-Hill Book Co, 1971.

40. *Architects Handbook of Professional Practice.* Washington DC, The American Institute of Architects, 1972-.

41. Packard RT, AIA, (ed): *Architectural Graphic Standards,* ed 7. New York, John Wiley and Sons, 1981.

42. Dibner DR: *Your Architects Compensation.* Washington DC, The American Institute of Architects, 1978.

43. Callender JH (ed): *Time-Saver Standards for Architectural Design Data,* ed 6. New York, McGraw-Hill Book Co, 1982.

44. DeChiara J, Callender JH (eds): *Time-Saver Standards for Building Types,* ed 2. New York, McGraw-Hill Book Co, 1980.

45. McHugh RC: *Working Drawings Handbook.* New York, Van Nostrand Reinhold, 1983.

46. Stein JS: *Construction Glossary: An Encyclopedia Reference and Manual.* New York, John Wiley and Sons, 1980.

47. Lathrop JK (ed): *Life Safety Code Handbook.* Quincy, Mass, National Fire Protection Association, Inc.

48. *The CSI Manual of Practice.* Construction Specification Institute, Washington, DC.

49. Rosen HJ: *Principles of Specification Writing.* New York, Reinhold Publishing Corp, 1967.

50. *Determining Hospital Space Requirements—Space Guidelines Study.* Washington, DC, American Institute of Architects, 1984.

Appendix A

GLOSSARY OF
CONSTRUCTION INDUSTRY TERMS
with Particular Emphasis on Use in AIA Documents

1982
THE AMERICAN INSTITUTE OF ARCHITECTS

The American Institute of Architects first published a glossary in the 1963 Edition of Chapter 2, "The Construction Industry," of the *Architect's Handbook of Professional Practice*, identifying terms which are used in, or are special to, the construction industry.

In 1970, the glossary was completely rewritten and considerably expanded, and was published separately as the first comprehensive AIA *Glossary of Construction Industry Terms* used by, and applicable to, the construction industry.

The latest edition of the glossary has been further reviewed, revised and expanded to make it current and compatible with usage in the AIA practice documents and the construction industry.

Terms used in the AIA practice documents have been defined as used in those documents. This glossary is a helpful adjunct to their utilization and understanding. Consistent with the practice followed in the AIA documents, terms specifically defined in the documents are capitalized.

The principles followed in the selection of the terms found in the glossary were, first, to include those which have a special relationship, meaning or importance in the design professions, and the construction industry and, second, to exclude those which are self-explanatory or which are adequately defined in standard dictionaries.

Following these principles, more terms were rejected than included in order to make the glossary more manageable and useful—not only to those in the construction industry for whom it will be a valuable ready reference source, but also to those government agencies, attorneys, jurists, students and laymen who will have the need for occasional reference to an authoritative source of construction industry definitions. The failure of a particular term to be included does not imply that such term does not have a recognized meaning.

188

A

ACCEPTANCE: See **FINAL ACCEPTANCE**

ACCIDENT (insurance terminology): An unexpected event identifiable as to time and place resulting in personal injury or property damage. See also **OCCURRENCE.**

ADDENDUM: A written or graphic instrument issued by the Architect prior to the execution of the Contract which modifies or interprets the Bidding Documents by additions, deletions, clarifications or corrections. An addendum becomes part of the Contract Documents when the Contract is executed. Plural—**ADDENDA.** (Ref: AIA Documents A201, A501 and A701, and Handbook Chapter B-6.)

ADDITION: (1, to Contract Sum) Amount added to the Contract Sum by Change Order. See also **EXTRA.** (2, to a structure) A construction Project physically connected to an existing structure, as distinct from alterations within an existing structure. (3, to Contract Time) Extension of the Contract Time authorized by Change Order. (4, to the Work) Increase to the scope of Work included in the Contract authorized by Change Order.

ADDITIONAL SERVICES (of the Architect): Professional services which may, if authorized or confirmed in writing by the Owner, be rendered by the Architect in addition to the Basic Services or Designated Services identified in the Owner-Architect Agreement. (Ref: AIA Documents B141, B151, B161, B171, and B181, and Handbook Chapter D-1.)

ADDITIVE ALTERNATE: An alternate bid resulting in an addition to the same bidder's Base Bid. See also **ALTERNATE BID.**

ADMINISTRATION OF THE CONSTRUCTION CONTRACT: See **CONSTRUCTION PHASE—ADMINISTRATION OF THE CONSTRUCTION CONTRACT.**

ADVERTISEMENT FOR BIDS: Published public notice soliciting bids for a construction project or designated portion thereof, included as part of the Bidding Documents. Most frequently used to conform to legal requirements pertaining to projects to be constructed under public authority, and usually published in newspapers of general circulation in those political subdivisions from which the public funds are derived. See also **INVITATION TO BID.** (Ref. AIA Document A501.)

AGENCY: (1) Relationship between agent and principal. (2) Organization acting as agent. (3) Administrative subdivision of an organization, particularly in government.

AGENT: One authorized by another to act in the other's stead or behalf.

AGREEMENT: (1) A meeting of minds. (2) A legally enforceable promise or promises between two or among several persons. (3) On a construction project, the document stating the essential terms of the Contract between Owner and Contractor which incorporates by reference the other Contract Documents. (4) The document setting forth the terms of the Contract between the Architect and Owner or between the Architect and a consultant. **AGREEMENT** and **CONTRACT** are frequently used interchangeably without any intended change in meaning. See also (1) **FORM OF AGREEMENT;** (2) **CONTRACT.** (Ref: AIA Documents A101, A107, A111, A117, B141, B151, B161, B171, B181, C141 and C161, and Handbook Chapters D-1, D-2 and D-4.)

AGREEMENT FORM: See **FORM OF AGREEMENT.**

ALLOWANCE: See (1) **CASH ALLOWANCE;** (2) **CONTINGENCY ALLOWANCE.**

ALL RISK INSURANCE: Insurance against loss arising from any cause other than those perils or causes specifically excluded by name. This contrasts with the ordinary type of policy which names the peril or perils insured against. See **PROPERTY INSURANCE.**

ALTERATIONS: (1) A construction project (or portion of a project) comprising revisions within or to prescribed elements of an existing structure, as distinct from additions to an existing structure. (2) Remodeling. See also **ADDITION.**

ALTERNATE BID: Amount stated in the bid to be added to or deducted from the amount of the Base Bid if the corresponding change in the Work, as described in the Bidding Documents, is accepted. (Ref: AIA Document A501 and Handbook Chapter B-6.)

APPLICATION FOR PAYMENT: Contractor's certified request for payment of amount due for completed portions of the Work and, if the Contract so provides, for materials or equipment delivered and suitably stored pending their incorporation into the Work. (Ref: AIA Documents A101, A107, A201, G702 and G703, and Handbook Chapter B-7.)

APPRAISAL: See **COST APPRAISAL.**

APPROVAL, ARCHITECT'S: Architect's written or imprinted acknowledgement that materials, equipment or methods of construction are acceptable for use in the Work, or accepting a Contractor's or Owner's request or claim as valid.

APPROVED EQUAL: Material, equipment or method approved by the Architect for use in the Work as being acceptable as an equivalent in essential attributes to the material, equipment or method specified in the Contract Documents. (Ref: Handbook Chapters B-6 and D-4.)

ARBITRATION: Method of settling claims or disputes between parties to a Contract, rather than by litigation, under which an arbitrator or a panel of arbitrators, selected for specialized knowledge in the field in question, hears the evidence and renders a decision. (Ref: Construction Industry Arbitration Rules of the American Arbitration Association and AIA Documents A107, A117, A177, A201, B141, B151, B161, B171, B181, B727, C141 and C161, and Handbook Chapter B-3).

ARCHITECT: Designation reserved, usually by law, for a person or organization professionally qualified and duly licensed to perform architectural services, including but not necessarily limited to analysis of Project requirements, creation and development of the Project design, preparation of Drawings, Specifications and bidding requirements, and general Administration of the Construction Contract.

ARCHITECT-ENGINEER: An individual or firm offering professional services as both architect and engineer.

ARCHITECT-IN-TRAINING: See **INTERN ARCHITECT.**

ARCHITECTURAL AREA OF BUILDINGS: The sum of the adjusted areas of the several floors of a building, computed in accordance with AIA Document D101. See **AREA METHOD.** See also **STANDARD NET ASSIGNABLE AREA.** (Ref: AIA Document D101 and Handbook Chapter B-5.)

ARCHITECTURAL VOLUME OF BUILDINGS: The sum of the products of the architectural areas of a building (using the area of a single story for multistory portions having the same area on each floor) and the height from the underside of the lowest floor construction system to the average height of the surface of the finished roof above the various parts of the building. See **ARCHITECTURAL AREA OF BUILDINGS.** (Ref: AIA Document D101 and Handbook Chapter B-5.)

AREA METHOD (of estimating cost): Method of estimating Probable Construction Cost by multiplying the architectural area by an estimated current cost per unit area. See **ARCHITECTURAL AREA OF BUILDINGS.** See also **ARCHITECTURAL VOLUME OF BUILDINGS** and **VOLUME METHOD.** (Ref: AIA Document D101 and Handbook Chapter B-5.)

ARTICLE: In the AIA documents, the primary division of a document.

AS-BUILT DRAWINGS: See **RECORD DRAWINGS.**

ASSOCIATE (of an office or firm): A member of an Architect's staff who has a special employment arrangement. (Ref: Handbook Chapter B-1.)

ASSOCIATE (or **ASSOCIATED**) **ARCHITECT:** An Architect who has a temporary arrangement with another Architect to collaborate in the performance of services for a specific project or series of projects. See also **JOINT VENTURE.** (Ref: Handbook Chapters B-1 and D-2.)

ASSUMED LIABILITY: Liability which arises from an agreement between people, as opposed to liability which arises from common or statutory law. See also **CONTRACTUAL LIABILITY.**

ATTORNEY-IN-FACT: A person authorized to act for or in behalf of another person or entity, to the extent usually prescribed in a written instrument known as a power of attorney. See also **POWER OF ATTORNEY**. (Ref: Handbook Chapter B-2.)

AUTOMATIC REINSTATEMENT: A provision in an insurance policy that will automatically return the amount of insurance to its original amount after a loss has been paid or property restored. When a policy does not contain this provision, the original amount is usually reduced by the amount of loss paid.

AWARD: See **CONTRACT AWARD**.

AXONOMETRIC DRAWING: A perspective drawing showing plan and partial elevations on the same drawing. The plan is rotated from the picture plane and lines are projected vertically from the plan to form partial elevations. See also **ISOMETRIC DRAWING**.

B

BASE BID SPECIFICATIONS: The specifications listing or describing only those materials, equipment, and methods of construction upon which the Bid must be predicated, exclusive of any Alternate Bids. See also (1) **SPECIFICATIONS**; (2) **CLOSED SPECIFICATIONS**. (Ref: Handbook Chapter D-4.)

BASE BID SUM: Amount of money stated in the Bid as the sum for which the bidder offers to perform the Work described in the Bidding Documents, prior to adjustments for Alternate Bids which are also submitted. (Ref: Handbook Chapter D-4.)

BASIC SERVICES (of the Architect): The Architect's Basic Services consist of the Phases described in the Owner-Architect Agreement. (Ref: AIA Documents B141, B151, B171, B181, and B727 and Handbook Chapter D-1.)

BENEFICIAL OCCUPANCY: Use of a project or portion thereof for the purpose intended. See also **DATE OF SUBSTANTIAL COMPLETION**.

BENEFITS, MANDATORY & CUSTOMARY: Personnel benefits required by law (such as employment taxes and other statutory employee benefits), and by custom (such as insurance, sick leave, holidays, vacations, pensions and similar contributions and benefits).

BID: A complete and properly signed proposal to do the Work or designated portion thereof for the amount or amounts stipulated therein; submitted in accordance with the Bidding Documents. (Ref: AIA Document A501 and Handbook Chapter D-4.)

BID BOND: Form of bid security executed by the bidder as Principal and by a Surety to guarantee that the bidder will enter into a contract within a specified time and furnish any required Performance Bond, and Labor and Material Payment Bond. See also (1) **BID SECURITY**; (2) **SURETY**. (Ref: AIA Document A310 and Handbook Chapter B-2.)

BID DATE: The date established by the Owner or the Architect for the receipt of Bids. See also **BID TIME**. (Ref: AIA Document A501 and Handbook Chapter D-4.)

BID FORM: A form furnished to a bidder to be completed, signed and submitted as the bidder's Bid. (Ref: AIA Documents A501 and A701, and Handbook Chapters D-4 and D-5.)

BID GUARANTEE: See **BID SECURITY**.

BID LETTING: See **BID OPENING**.

BID OPENING: The opening and tabulation of Bids submitted within the prescribed bid time and in conformity with the prescribed procedures. Preferable to **BID LETTING**. See also **BID TIME**.

BID PRICE: The amount stated in the Bid for which the bidder offers to perform the Work.

BID SECURITY: The deposit of cash, certified check, cashier's check, bank draft, stocks/bonds, money order or Bid Bond submitted with a Bid and serving to guarantee to the Owner that the bidder, if awarded the Contract, will execute such Contract in accordance with the requirements of the Bidding Documents. (Ref: AIA Document A501.)

BID TIME: The date and hour established by the Owner or the Architect for the receipt of Bids. See also **BID DATE**. (Ref: AIA Document A501 and Handbook Chapter D-4.)

BIDDER: A person or entity who submits a Bid, generally one who submits a Bid for a prime contract with the Owner, as distinct from a sub-bidder who submits a Bid to a prime bidder. Technically, a bidder is not a contractor on a specific project until a contract exists between the bidder and the Owner. (Ref: AIA Document A501 and Handbook Chapter D-4.)

BIDDER, SELECTED: See **SELECTED BIDDER.**

BIDDERS, INVITED: See **INVITED BIDDERS.**

BIDDING DOCUMENTS: The Advertisement or Invitation to Bid, Instructions to Bidders, the bid form, other sample bidding and contract forms, and the proposed Contract Documents including any Addenda issued prior to receipt of Bids. (Ref: AIA Documents A501 and A701.)

BIDDING OR NEGOTIATION PHASE: The Phase of the Architect's Services during which competitive bids or negotiated proposals are sought as the basis for awarding a contract. (Ref: AIA Documents B141, B151, B162, B181 and D200, and Handbook Chapters D-1 and D-4.)

BIDDING PERIOD: The calendar period beginning at the time of issuance of Bidding Documents and ending at the prescribed bid time. See also **BID TIME.**

BIDDING REQUIREMENTS: See **BIDDING DOCUMENTS.** (Ref: AIA Documents A501 and A701.)

BILL OF QUANTITIES: See **QUANTITY SURVEY.**

BILL OF SALE: A document executed by the seller or other transferor of property by which the transferor's ownership or other interest in tangible property is transferred to the buyer or other transferee. Title frequently passes by delivery, affixation or other acts of the parties. A bill of sale is often merely confirmatory of the transfer. Frequently it must be notarized to satisfy regulatory requirements.

BODILY INJURY (insurance terminology): Physical injury, sickness or disease sustained by a person. See also **PERSONAL INJURY.**

BOILER AND MACHINERY INSURANCE: Special insurance covering steam boilers, other pressure vessels and related equipment and machinery. This insurance covers damage or injury to property resulting from explosion of steam boilers which is not covered by extended coverage perils. (Ref: AIA Document A201 and Handbook Chapter B-2.)

BONA FIDE BID: Bid submitted in good faith, complete and in accordance with the Bidding Documents, and properly signed by a person legally authorized to sign such Bid. (Ref: Handbook Chapters D-1 and D-4.)

BOND: See (1) **BID BOND;** (2) **COMPLETION BOND;** (3) **FIDELITY BOND;** (4) **LABOR AND MATERIAL PAYMENT BOND;** (5) **PERFORMANCE BOND;** (6) **STATUTORY BOND;** (7) **SURETY BOND.**

BONUS AND PENALTY CLAUSE: A provision in the Contract for payment of a bonus to the Contractor for completing the Work prior to a stipulated date, and a charge against the Contractor for failure to complete the Work by such stipulated date.

BONUS CLAUSE: A provision in the Construction Contract for additional payment to the Contractor as a reward for completing the Work prior to a stipulated date. (Ref: Handbook Chapter D-5.)

BOUNDARY SURVEY: A mathematically closed diagram of the complete peripheral boundary of a site, reflecting dimensions, compass bearings and angles. It should bear a licensed land surveyor's signed certification, and may include a metes and bounds or other written description.

BREAKDOWN, CONTRACTOR'S: See **SCHEDULE OF VALUES.**

BUDGET, CONSTRUCTION: The sum established by the Owner as available for construction of the Project, including contingencies for bidding and for changes during construction.

BUDGET, PROJECT: The sum established by the Owner as available for the entire Project, including the construction budget, land costs, equipment costs, financing costs, compensation for professional services, costs of Owner-furnished goods and services, contingency allowance, and other similar established or estimated costs. (Ref: Handbook Chapter B-5.)

BUILDER'S RISK INSURANCE: A specialized form of property insurance which provides coverage for loss or damage to the Work during the course of construction. See also (1) **PROPERTY INSURANCE;** (2) **ALL RISK INSURANCE.** (Ref: Handbook Chapter B-2.)

BUILDING CODE: See **CODES.**

BUILDING INSPECTOR: A representative of a governmental authority employed to inspect construction for compliance of applicable codes, regulations and ordinances. (Ref: Handbook Chapter B-7.)

BUILDING PERMIT: A permit issued by appropriate governmental authority allowing construction of a project in accordance with approved Drawings and Specifications.

BULLETIN: A document issued by the Architect after contract award which may include Drawings and other information used to solicit a proposal for a change in the Work. A bulletin becomes part of the Contract Documents only after being incorporated in a Change Order. Sometimes called a **REQUEST FOR A CHANGE.**

C

CARE, CUSTODY AND CONTROL (insurance terminology): The term used to describe a standard exclusion in liability insurance policies. Under this exclusion, the liability insurance does not apply to damage to property over which the insured is for any purpose exercising physical control.

CASH ALLOWANCE: An amount established in the Contract Documents for inclusion in the Contract Sum to cover the cost of prescribed items not specified in detail, with provision that variations between such amount and the finally determined cost of the prescribed items will be reflected in Change Orders appropriately adjusting the Contract Sum. (Ref: AIA Document A201.)

CASH DISCOUNT: The amount which can be deducted from a seller's invoice for payment within a stipulated period of time.

CERTIFICATE FOR PAYMENT: A statement from the Architect to the Owner confirming the amount of money due the Contractor for Work accomplished or materials and equipment suitably stored, or both. (Ref: AIA Documents A101, A201, B141 and G702, and Handbook Chapter D-6.)

CERTIFICATE OF INSURANCE: A document issued by an authorized representative of an insurance company stating the types, amounts and effective dates of insurance in force for a designated insured. (Ref: AIA Documents A201 and G705.)

CERTIFICATE OF OCCUPANCY: Document issued by governmental authority certifying that all or a designated portion of a building complies with the provisions of applicable statutes and regulations, and permitting occupancy for its designated use. (Ref: Handbook Chapter B-7.)

CERTIFICATE OF SUBSTANTIAL COMPLETION: A certificate prepared by the Architect on the basis of an inspection stating that the Work or a designated portion thereof is substantially complete, which establishes the Date of Substantial Completion; states the responsibilities of the Owner and the Contractor for security, maintenance, heat, utilities, damage to the Work, and insurance; and fixes the time within which the Contractor shall complete the items listed therein. See **DATE OF SUBSTANTIAL COMPLETION.** (Ref: AIA Documents A201 and G704.)

CHANGE ORDER: A written order to the Contractor signed by the Owner and the Architect, issued after the execution of the Contract, authorizing a change in the Work or an adjustment in the Contract Sum or the Contract Time. The Contract Sum and the Contract Time may be changed only by Change Order. A Change Order signed by the Contractor indicates the Contractor's agreement therewith, including the adjustment in the Contract Sum or the Contract Time. (Ref: AIA Document A201 and Handbook Chapter D-3.)

CHANGES IN THE WORK: Changes ordered by the Owner within the general scope of the Contract, consisting of additions, deletions, or other revisions, the Contract Sum and the Contract Time being adjusted accordingly. All such changes in the Work shall be authorized by Change Order, and shall be performed under the applicable conditions of the Contract Documents. See also **MINOR CHANGES IN THE WORK.** (Ref: AIA Documents A201 and G701, and Handbook Chapter B-7.)

CLARIFICATION DRAWING: A graphic interpretation of the Drawings or other Contract Documents issued by the Architect.

CLAUSE: In the AIA Documents, a subdivision of a Subparagraph, identified by four numerals, e.g., 2.2.10.1.

CLERK OF THE WORKS: Variously used to mean **OWNER'S INSPECTOR** or Owner's site representative.

CLOSED LIST OF BIDDERS: See **INVITED BIDDERS.**

CLOSED SPECIFICATIONS: Specifications stipulating the use of specific or proprietary products or processes without provision for substitution. See also **BASE BID SPECIFICATIONS.**

CODES: Regulations, ordinances or statutory requirements of a governmental unit relating to building construction and occupancy, adopted and administered for the protection of the public health, safety and welfare.

COINSURANCE: An insurance policy provision which requires the insured to carry insurance equal to a named percentage of the value of the property covered, or share in the loss proportionately in event of a claim.

COLLAPSE INSURANCE: Insurance to cover building and contents loss or damaged caused by collapse.

COMPENSATION: (1) Payment for services rendered or products or materials furnished or delivered. (2) Payment in satisfaction of claims for damages suffered.

COMPLETED OPERATIONS INSURANCE: Liability insurance coverage for injuries to persons or damage to property occurring after an operation is completed (1) when all operations under the Contract have been completed or abandoned; or (2) when all operations at one project site are completed; or (3) when the portion of the Work out of which the injury or damage arises has been put to its intended use by the person or organization for whom that portion of the Work was done. Completed Operations Insurance does not apply to damage to the completed Work itself.

COMPLETED VALUE FORM PROPERTY INSURANCE: See **PROPERTY INSURANCE.**

COMPLETION BOND: Bond of the Contractor or the Owner in which a surety guarantees to the lender that the Project will be completed free of liens.

COMPLETION DATE: See **DATE OF SUBSTANTIAL COMPLETION.** (Ref: Handbook Chapter D-5.)

COMPLETION LIST: See **INSPECTION LIST.**

COMPREHENSIVE AUTOMOBILE LIABILITY INSURANCE: Insurance covering claims for bodily injury or property damage arising from the ownership, maintenance, or use of any automobile, owned or nonowned.

COMPREHENSIVE GENERAL LIABILITY INSURANCE: A broad form of liability insurance covering claims for bodily injury and property damage which combines under one policy coverage for all liability exposures (except those specially excluded) on a blanket basis and automatically covers new and unknown hazards that may develop. Comprehensive General Liability Insurance automatically includes contractual liability coverage for certain types of contracts. Products Liability, Completed Operations Liability and broader Contractual Liability coverages are available on an optional basis. This policy may also be written to include Automobile Liability.

COMPREHENSIVE SERVICES: Professional services performed by the Architect including traditional services and such other services as project analysis, programming, land use studies, feasibility investigations, financing, construction management and special consulting services. (Ref: AIA Document B161 and B162.)

CONDITIONS OF THE CONTRACT: Those portions of the Contract Documents which define the rights and responsibilities of the contracting parties and of others involved in the Work. The Conditions of the Contract include General Conditions, Supplementary Conditions and other Conditions.

CONSENT OF SURETY: Written consent of the surety on a Performance Bond and/or Labor and Material Payment Bond to such Contract changes as Change Orders or reductions in the Contractor's retainage, or to final payment, or to waiving notification of Contract changes. The term is also used with respect to an extension of time in a Bid Bond. (Ref: AIA Documents A310, A311 and G707.)

CONSEQUENTIAL LOSS: Loss not directly caused by damage to property, but which may arise as a result of such damage—e.g., damage to other portions of a building or its contents due to roof leaks.

CONSTRUCTION COST (for calculating compensation to the Architect): The total cost or estimated cost to the Owner of all elements of the Project designed or specified by the Architect, including at current market rates (with a reasonable allowance for overhead and profit) the cost of labor and materials furnished by the Owner and any equipment which has been designed, specified, selected or specially provided for by the Architect, but not including the compensation of the Architect and the Architect's consultants, the cost of land, rights-of-way, or other costs which are the responsibility of the Owner. (Ref: AIA Document B141.)

CONSTRUCTION DOCUMENTS: Drawings and Specifications setting forth in detail the requirements for the construction of the Project. (Ref: Handbook Chapters B-6 and D-4.)

CONSTRUCTION DOCUMENTS PHASE: The Phase of the Architect's Services in which the Architect prepares from the approved Design Development Documents, the Construction Documents and assists the Owner in the preparation of the Bidding Documents. (Ref: AIA Documents B141, B151, B162, B181 and D200, and Handbook Chapters B-4 and D-1.)

CONSTRUCTION INSPECTOR: See **INSPECTOR**.

CONSTRUCTION MANAGEMENT: Special management services provided to an Owner by an Architect or other person or entity possessing requisite training and experience during the Design Phase and/or Construction Phase of a Project. Such management services may include advice on the time and cost consequences of design and construction decisions, scheduling, cost control, coordination of contract negotiations and awards, timely purchasing of critical materials and long-lead items and coordination of construction activities. (Ref: AIA Documents A101/CM, A201/CM, A311/CM, A511/CM, B141/CM, B161/CM and B801.)

CONSTRUCTION MANAGER: As used in AIA Documents, the term refers to an individual or entity who provides construction management services with a fiduciary duty to the Owner for both the Design Phase and/or Construction Phase of a Project. As used in other contexts in the construction industry, it may refer only to a commercial, arms-length relationship between an Owner and Construction Manager, or a combination of a fiduciary and commercial relationship over the life of a Project. See also **CONSTRUCTION MANAGEMENT**. (Ref: AIA Documents B141/CM, B161/CM and B801.)

CONSTRUCTION PHASE-ADMINISTRATION OF THE CONSTRUCTION CONTRACT: The Phase of the Architect's Services which includes the Architect's general administration of the Construction Contract(s). See also **CONTRACT ADMINISTRATION**. (Ref: AIA Document A201, B141, B151, B162, B181 and D200, and Handbook Chapters B-2, B-3, B-7, D-1 and D-3.)

CONSULTANT: A person or entity who provides professional advice or services.

CONTINGENCY ALLOWANCE: A sum included in the Project budget designated to cover unpredictble or unforeseen items of Work, or changes in the Work subsequently required by the Owner. See **BUDGET, PROJECT**. (Ref: Handbook Chapter D-4.)

CONTINGENT AGREEMENT: An agreement, generally between an Owner and an Architect, in which some portion of the Architect's compensation is contingent upon the Owner's obtaining funds for the Project (such as by successful referendum, sale of bonds or securing of other financing), or upon some other specially prescribed condition.

CONTINGENT LIABILITY: (1) Liability which is not absolute and fixed, but is dependent upon the occurrence of some uncertain future event or the existence of an uncertain specified condition. (2) Particularly in insurance law, liability imposed upon an individual or entity because of injuries or damages caused by persons or entities, other than employees, for whose acts or omissions the first party may be legally responsible.

CONTRACT: A legally enforceable promise or agreement between two or among several persons. See also **AGREEMENT**.

CONTRACT ADMINISTRATION: The duties and responsibilities of the Architect during the Construction Phase. (Ref: AIA Documents A201, B141, B151, B161, B162, B171, B181 and B352, and Handbook Chapter B-7.)

CONTRACT AWARD: A communication from an Owner accepting a bid or negotiated proposal. An award creates legal obligations between the parties. (Ref: AIA Document A501 and Handbook Chapter D-4.)

CONTRACT DATE: See **DATE OF AGREEMENT**.

CONTRACT DOCUMENTS: The Owner-Contractor Agreement, the Conditions of the Contract (General, Supplementary and other Conditions), the Drawings, the Specifications, and all Addenda issued prior to and all Modifications issued after execution of the Contract; and any other items that may be specifically stipulated as being included in the Contract Documents. (Ref: AIA Document A201 and Handbook Chapters B-7 and D-3.)

CONTRACT LIMIT: A limit line or perimeter line established on the Drawings or elsewhere in the Contract Documents defining the boundaries of the site available to the Contractor for construction purposes.

CONTRACT SUM: The sum stated in the Owner-Contractor Agreement, which is the total amount payable by the Owner to the Contractor for the performance of the Work under the Contract Documents. The Contract Sum may be adjusted only by Change Order. (Ref: AIA Document A201 and Handbook Chapter D-5.)

CONTRACT TIME: The period of time allotted in the Contract Documents for Substantial Completion of the Work, including authorized adjustments thereto. The Contract Time may be adjusted only by Change Order. (Ref: AIA Document A201 and Handbook Chapter D-5.)

CONTRACTING OFFICER: The person designated as the official representative of the Owner with specific authority to act in the Owner's behalf in connection with a Project. In the federal, and many state and local procurement systems, the **CONTRACTING OFFICER** has authority to decide disputes, either finally or subject to review procedures. See also **OWNER'S REPRESENTATIVE.**

CONTRACTOR: (1) One who contracts. (2) In construction terminology, the person or entity responsible for performing the Work and identified as such in the Owner-Contractor Agreement. (Ref: Handbook Chapter D-5.)

CONTRACTOR'S AFFIDAVIT: A certified statement of the Contractor, properly notarized, relating to payment of debts and claims, release of liens, or similar matters requiring specific evidence for the protection of the Owner. See also **NONCOLLUSION AFFIDAVIT.** (Ref: AIA Documents G706 and G706A.)

CONTRACTOR'S LIABILITY INSURANCE: Insurance purchased and maintained by the Contractor to protect the Contractor from specified claims which may arise out of or result from the Contractor's operations under the Contract, whether such operations are by the Contractor or by any Subcontractor or by anyone directly or indirectly employed by any of them, or by anyone for whose acts any of them may be liable. (Ref: AIA Documents A201 and G705, and Handbook Chapter B-2.)

CONTRACTOR'S OPTION: Provision of the Contract Documents under which the Contractor may select certain specified materials, methods or systems at the Contractor's own option, without change in the Contract Sum. (Ref: Handbook Chapters B-6 and D-4.)

CONTRACTUAL LIABILITY: Liability assumed by a person or entity under a contract. "Indemnification" or "hold harmless" clauses are examples of contractual liability. (Ref: AIA Documents A201 and G705.)

COST APPRAISAL: Evaluation or estimate (preferably by a qualified professional appraiser) of the market or other value, cost, utility, or other attribute of land or other facility.

COST BREAKDOWN: See **SCHEDULE OF VALUES.**

COST PLUS FEE AGREEMENT: An Agreement under which the Contractor (in an Owner-Contractor Agreement) or the Architect (in an Owner-Architect Agreement) is reimbursed for the direct and indirect costs of performance of the Agreement and, in addition, is paid a fee for services. The fee is usually stated as a stipulated sum or as a percentage of cost. (Ref: AIA Documents A111, A117, B141 and B161.)

CRITICAL PATH METHOD (CPM): A charting of all events and operations to be encountered in completing a given process, rendered in a form permitting determination of the relative significance of each event, and establishing the optimum sequence and duration of operations. See also **PERT SCHEDULE.** (Ref: Handbook Chapter B-7.)

CUBAGE: See **ARCHITECTURAL VOLUME OF BUILDINGS.**

D

DATE OF AGREEMENT: The date stated in the Agreement. If no date is stated, it could be the date on which the Agreement is actually signed, if this is recorded, or it may be the date established by the award.

DATE OF COMMENCEMENT OF THE WORK: The date established in a notice to the Contractor to proceed or, in the absence of such notice, the date of the Owner-Contractor Agreement or such other date as may be established therein. (Ref: AIA Document A201 and Handbook Chapters B-3, D-3 and D-5.)

DATE OF SUBSTANTIAL COMPLETION: The Date certified by the Architect when the Work or a designated portion thereof is sufficiently complete, in accordance with the Contract Documents, so the Owner can occupy the Work or designated portion thereof for the use for which it is intended. (Ref: AIA Documents A201 and G704, and Handbook Chapters B-7 and D-3.)

DEDUCTION (from Contract Sum): Amount deducted from the Contract Sum by Change Order.

DEDUCTIVE ALTERNATE: An Alternate Bid resulting in a deduction from the Base Bid of the same Bidder. See also **ALTERNATE BID.**

DEFECTIVE WORK: The Work not conforming with the Contract requirements. See also **NONCONFORMING WORK.**

DEFICIENCIES: See **DEFECTIVE WORK.**

DEPOSIT FOR BIDDING DOCUMENTS: Monetary deposit required to obtain a set of Bidding Documents. (Ref: AIA Documents A501 and A701, and Handbook Chapters B-6 and D-4.)

DESIGNATED SERVICES (of the Architect): Those services necessary to the Project agreed to be performed directly by the Architect, or through the Architect by utilization of outside services, and by coordination services performed by the Architect on services provided by the Owner. (Ref: AIA Documents B161 and B162.)

DESIGN-BUILD PROCESS: A process in which a person or entity assumes responsibility under a single contract for both the design and construction of the Project. (Ref: Handbook Chapter A-2.)

DESIGN DEVELOPMENT DOCUMENTS: Drawings and other documents which fix and describe the size and character of the entire Project as to architectural, structural, mechanical and electrical systems, materials and such other elements as may be appropriate. (Ref: AIA Documents B141, B162 and B171.)

DESIGN DEVELOPMENT PHASE: The Phase of the Architect's Services in which the Architect prepares from the approved Schematic Design Studies, for approval by the Owner, the Design Development Documents, and submits to the Owner a further Statement of Probable Construction Cost. (Ref: AIA Documents B141, B162, B171 and D200.)

DESIGN PROFESSIONS: See **ENVIRONMENTAL DESIGN PROFESSIONS.**

DETAIL: A drawing, at a larger scale, of a part of another drawing, indicating in detail the design, location, composition and correlation of the elements and materials shown. (Ref: Handbook Chapter B-6.)

DIAGRAM: A schematic representation of a Project system, subsystem or portion thereof. See also **DRAWINGS.**

DIRECT EXPENSE: All items of expense directly incurred by or attributable to a specific project, assignment or task.

DIRECT PERSONNEL EXPENSE: Direct salaries of all the Architect's personnel engaged on the Project, and the portion of the cost of their mandatory and customary contributions and benefits related thereto.

DIRECT SALARY EXPENSE: Direct salaries of all the Architect's personnel engaged on the Project, but excluding the cost of contributions and benefits related thereto, whether mandatory or customary.

DIVISION (of the Specifications): One of the sixteen basic organizational subdivisions used in the Uniform Construction Index. (Ref: Handbook Chapter B-6.)

DOCUMENT DEPOSIT: See **DEPOSIT FOR BIDDING DOCUMENTS.**

DRAWINGS: Graphic and pictorial documents showing the design, location and dimensions of the elements of a Project. Drawings generally include plans, elevations, sections, details, schedules and diagrams. When capitalized, the term refers to the graphic and pictorial portions of the Contract Documents. (Ref: Handbook Chapter B-6.)

DUE CARE: A legal term indicating the requirement for a professional to exercise reasonable care, skill, ability and judgment under the circumstances. Performance of duties and services must be consistent with the level of reasonable care, skill, ability and judgment provided by reputable professionals in the same geographical area and at the same period of time. Failure to exercise **DUE CARE** constitutes **NEGLIGENCE.**

E

ELEVATION: (1) A two-dimensional graphic representation of the design, location and dimensions of the Project, or parts thereof, seen in a vertical plane viewed from a given direction. See also **DRAWINGS.** (2) Distance above or below a prescribed datum or reference point. (Ref: Handbook Chapter B-6.)

EMPLOYER'S LIABILITY INSURANCE: Insurance protection for the employer against claims by employees or employees' dependents for damages which arise out of injuries or diseases sustained in the course of their work, and which are based on common law negligence rather than on liability under workers' compensation acts.

ENGINEER: See **PROFESSIONAL ENGINEER.**

ENGINEER-IN-TRAINING: (sometimes called Engineer Intern). Designation for a person qualified for professional engineering registration in all respects except the required professional experience and successful completion of an examination on the principles of practice.

ENGINEERING OFFICER: A person designated, usually by a military component or a corporation, as having authoritative charge over certain specific enginering operations and duties.

ENVIRONMENTAL DESIGN PROFESSIONS: The professions collectively responsible for the design of man's physical environment, including architecture, engineering, landscape architecture, urban planning and similar environment-related professions.

ERRATUM: Correction of a printing, typographical or editorial error. Not to be confused with **ADDENDUM.** Plural **ERRATA.**

ERRORS AND OMISSIONS INSURANCE: See **PROFESSIONAL LIABILITY INSURANCE.**

ESTIMATE: See (1) **BUDGET, PROJECT;** (2) **ESTIMATE** (Contractor's); (3) **ESTIMATE OF CONSTRUCTION COST, DETAILED;** (4) **STATEMENT OF PROBABLE CONSTRUCTION COST.**

ESTIMATE (Contractor's): (1) A forecast of Construction Cost, as opposed to a firm bid, prepared by a Contractor for a Project or a portion thereof. (2) A term sometimes used to denote a Contractor's application or request for a progress payment. With respect to (2), see also **APPLICATION FOR PAYMENT.**

ESTIMATE OF CONSTRUCTION COST, DETAILED: A forecast of Construction Cost prepared on the basis of a detailed analysis of materials and labor for all items of Work, as contrasted with an estimate based on current area, volume or similar unit costs. (Ref: Handbook Chapter B-5.)

EXCESS LIABILITY INSURANCE: Insurance providing excess liability coverage subject to the same terms and conditions as specified in the primary policy or policies. See also **UMBRELLA LIABILITY INSURANCE.**

EXECUTION OF THE CONTRACT (or AGREEMENT): (1) Performance of a **CONTRACT** or **AGREEMENT** according to its terms; (2) The acts of signing and delivering between the parties of the document or documents constituting the **CONTRACT** or **AGREEMENT.**

EXPERT WITNESS: A witness in a court case or other legal proceeding, who, by virtue of experience, training, skill and knowledge of a particular field or subject, is recognized as being especially qualified to render an informed opinion on matters relating to that field or subject.

EXPOSURE: Estimate of the probability of loss from some hazard, contingency or circumstance, such as proximity of insured property to adjoining property or lack of proximity to fire hydrants. Also used to signify the estimate of an insurer's liability under a policy from any one loss or accident.

EXPRESS WARRANTY: A warranty created or confirmed by affirmation of fact or promise made by the warrantor; any description of materials or equipment, or sample or model, furnished by or agreed to by the warrantor creates an express warranty.

EXTENDED COVERAGE INSURANCE: An endorsement to a property insurance policy which extends the perils covered to include windstorm, hail, riot, civil commotion, explosion (except steam boiler), air craft, vehicles and smoke. See (1) **PROPERTY INSURANCE;** (2) **BOILER & MACHINERY INSURANCE.**

EXTRA: A term sometimes used to denote an item of Work involving additional cost. See also **ADDITION** (to Contract Sum).

EXTRA SERVICES: See **ADDITIONAL SERVICES** (of the Architect).

F

FEASIBILITY STUDY: A detailed investigation and analysis conducted to determine the financial, economic, technical or other advisability of a proposed project.

FEE: A term used to denote compensation for professional ability, capability and availability of organization, excluding compensation for direct, indirect and/or reimbursable expenses, as an Agreement based on a "professional fee plus expenses." Sometimes used to denote compensation of any kind for services rendered. See also **COMPENSATION.** (Ref: AIA Documents A111, B141 and C141 and Handbook Chapters D-1 and D-2.)

FEE PLUS EXPENSE AGREEMENT: See **COST PLUS FEE AGREEMENT.**

FIDELITY BOND: A surety bond that reimburses an employer named in the bond for loss sustained by reason of the dishonest acts of an employee covered by the bond.

FIELD ENGINEER: Term used by certain governmental agencies to designate their representative at the Project site. See also **PROJECT REPRESENTATIVE.**

FIELD REPRESENTATIVE: See **PROJECT REPRESENTATIVE.**

FINAL ACCEPTANCE: The Owner's acceptance of the Project from the Contractor upon certification by the Architect of final completion. Final acceptance is confirmed by the making of final payment unless otherwise stipulated at the time of making such payment. (Ref: AIA Document A201 and Handbook Chapters B-7 and D-6.)

FINAL COMPLETION: Term denoting that the Work has been completed in accordance with the terms and conditions of the Contract Documents. (Ref: AIA Document A201 and Handbook Chapters B-7 and D-6.)

FINAL INSPECTION: Final review of the Project by the Architect to determine final completion, prior to issuance of the final Certificate for Payment. (Ref: AIA Document G703.)

FINAL PAYMENT: Payment made by the Owner to the Contractor, upon issuance by the Architect of the final Certificate for Payment, of the entire unpaid balance of the Contract Sum as adjusted by Change Orders. See also **FINAL ACCEPTANCE.** (Ref: AIA Document A201 and Handbook Chapters B-7 and D-6.)

FIRE AND EXTENDED COVERAGE INSURANCE: See **PROPERTY INSURANCE.**

FIXED LIMIT OF CONSTRUCTION COST: The maximum Construction Cost established in the Agreement between the Owner and the Architect. See also **BUDGET,** CONSTRUCTION and **CONSTRUCTION COST.** (Ref: AIA Documents B141, B151, B161 and B171.)

FORCE ACCOUNT: Term used when Work is ordered, often under urgent circumstances, to be performed without prior agreement as to lump sum or unit price cost thereof and is to be billed at the cost of labor, materials and equipment, insurance, taxes, etc., plus an agreed percentage for overhead and profit; sometimes used to describe work performed by Owner's own forces in a similar manner.

FORMAT (for Construction Specifications): Standardized arrangement for the Project Manual including bidding information, contract forms, Conditions of the Contract, and Specifications subdivided into sixteen Divisions.

FORM OF AGREEMENT: A document setting forth in printed form the general provisions of an agreement, with spaces provided for insertion of specific data relating to a particular Project. (Ref: AIA Documents A101, A107, A111, A117, B141, B151, B161, B171, B181 and B727 and Handbook Chapters D-1, D-2 and D-5.)

FOUNDATION EXCLUSION: A clause in a fire insurance policy stating that the policy does not insure foundations below ground level. As a result, their value is not used to determine the proper amount of insurance under a coinsurance clause.

G

GENERAL CONDITIONS (of the Contract for Construction): That part of the Contract Documents which sets forth many of the rights, responsibilities and relationships of the parties involved, particularly those provisions which are common to many construction projects. See also **CONDITIONS OF THE CONTRACT.** (Ref: AIA Documents A107, A117, A201 and A271 and Handbook Chapter D-3.)

GENERAL CONTRACT: (1) Under the single contract system, the Contract between the Owner and the Contractor for construction of the entire Work. (2) Under the separate contract system, a Contract between the Owner and a Contractor for general construction consisting of architectural and structural Work.

GENERAL REQUIREMENTS: Title of Division 1 of The Uniform Construction Index.

GUARANTEE: See WARRANTY.

GUARANTEED MAXIMUM COST: Sum established in an Agreement between Owner and Contractor as the maximum cost of performing specified Work on the basis of cost of labor and materials plus overhead expenses and profit. Preferable to GUARANTEED MAXIMUM PRICE (Ref: AIA Documents A111 and A117.)

GUARANTEED MAXIMUM PRICE: See GUARANTEED MAXIMUM COST.

GUARANTY: See WARRANTY.

GUARANTY BONDS: See (1) BID BOND; (2) COMPLETION BOND; (3) FIDELITY BOND; (4) LABOR AND MATERIAL PAYMENT BOND; (5) PERFORMANCE BOND; (6) SURETY BOND.

H

HEADING: A classification of related data used in the Filing System (Part Two of the Uniform Construction Index) as the first step in subdividing each of the sixteen Divisions and corresponding generally to the Sections used in Parts One, Three and Four.

HOLD HARMLESS: See INDEMNIFICATION. See also CONTRACTUAL LIABILITY.

I

IMPLIED WARRANTY: A warranty which exists, despite the absence of an express warranty, merely by reason of the factual situation and the conditions existing between the parties; usual implied warranties include (a) title to materials or equipment, (b) fitness for purpose, or (c) merchantable quality.

INCENTIVE CLAUSE: A term used to describe the savings which are shared proportionally in some agreed manner between an Owner and a Contractor and which are derived from the difference between the Guaranteed Maximum and the actual cost of a Project when the Work is performed on the basis of Cost Plus a Fee with a Guaranteed Maximum Cost. The terms of an Incentive Clause are normally included in the Agreement between the Owner and the Contractor.

INDEMNIFICATION: A contractual obligation by which one person or entity agrees to secure another against loss or damage from specified liabilities. See also CONTRACTUAL LIABILITY.

INDEMNIFICATION, IMPLIED: An indemnification which is implied by law rather than arising out of a contract to provide indemnification.

INDIRECT EXPENSE: Overhead expense; general office expense indirectly incurred and not directly related to a specific project. (Ref: Handbook Chapter B-1.)

INSPECTION: Examination of Work completed or in progress to determine its conformance with the requirements of the Contract Documents. The Architect ordinarily makes only two inspections of the Work, one to determine Substantial Completion, and the other to determine final completion. These inspections should be distinguished from the more general observations made by the Architect on visits to the site during the progress of the Work. The term is also used to mean examination of the work by a public official, Owner's representative, or others. (Ref: AIA Document A201 and Handbook Chapter B-7.)

INSPECTION LIST: A list of items of Work to be completed or corrected by the Contractor. Preferable to PUNCH LIST. (Ref: Handbook Chapter B-7.)

INSPECTOR: See (1) BUILDING INSPECTOR; (2) OWNER'S INSPECTOR; (3) RESIDENT ENGINEER.

INSTALLATION FLOATER: Insurance coverage for machinery and other prefabricated or preassembled equipment while it is being transported to the job site; this coverage continues until the items covered have been installed, tested and accepted.

INSTRUCTIONS TO BIDDERS: Instructions contained in the Bidding Documents for preparing and submitting bids for a construction Project or designated portion thereof. See also NOTICE TO BIDDERS. (Ref: AIA Documents A501 and A701, and Handbook Chapter D-4.)

INSURABLE INTEREST: Any interest in property or relation thereto of such a nature that damage to the property will cause pecuniary loss to the insured.

INSURABLE VALUE: The replacement cost of the Work at the site in the event of loss or damage caused by perils covered under the property insurance. The full insurable value of the Work at the site is usually determined as the Contract Sum less the cost of certain portions of the Work which are not subject to loss or damage caused by perils covered under the property insurance. See also **PROPERTY INSURANCE**. (Ref: AIA Document A201 and *Construction Bonds and Insurance Guide* published by AIA.)

INSURANCE: See (1) **ALL RISK INSURANCE**; (2) **BOILER AND MACHINERY INSURANCE**; (3) **BUILDER'S RISK INSURANCE**; (4) **COMPLETED OPERATIONS INSURANCE**; (5) **COMPREHENSIVE AUTOMOBILE LIABILITY INSURANCE**; (6) **COMPREHENSIVE GENERAL LIABILITY INSURANCE**; (7) **CONTRACTOR'S LIABILITY INSURANCE**; (8) **EMPLOYER'S LIABILITY INSURANCE**; (9) **EXCESS LIABILITY INSURANCE**; (10) **LIABILITY INSURANCE**; (11) **LOSS OF USE INSURANCE**; (12) **OWNER'S LIABILITY INSURANCE**; (13) **PROFESSIONAL LIABILITY INSURANCE**; (14) **PROPERTY DAMAGE INSURANCE**; (15) **PROPERTY INSURANCE**; (16) **PUBLIC LIABILITY INSURANCE**; (17) **SPECIAL HAZARDS INSURANCE**; (18) **UMBRELLA LIABILITY INSURANCE**; (19) **WORKERS' COMPENSATION INSURANCE**.

INTERN ARCHITECT: One pursuing a program of training in practice under the guidance of practicing Architects, with the objective of qualifying for registration as an Architect. Preferable to **ARCHITECT-IN-TRAINING**. (Ref: Handbook Chapter A-4.)

INVITATION TO BID: A portion of the Bidding Documents soliciting bids for a construction project. See also **ADVERTISEMENT FOR BIDS** and **NOTICE TO BIDDERS**. (Ref: AIA Document A501.)

INVITED BIDDERS: The bidders selected by the Owner, after consultation with the Architect, as the only ones from whom bids will be received. (Ref: AIA Document A501.)

ISOMETRIC DRAWING: A form of three-dimensional projection in which all of the principal planes are drawn parallel to corresponding established axes and at true dimensions. Horizontals are usually drawn at 30 degrees from the normal horizontal axes; verticals remain parallel to the normal vertical axis.

J

JOB CAPTAIN: The individual within the Architect's office normally responsible for preparation of the construction documents.

JOB SITE: See **SITE**.

JOB SUPERINTENDENT: See **SUPERINTENDENT**.

JOINT VENTURE: A collaborative undertaking by two or more persons or organizations for a specific Project or Projects, having the legal characteristics of a partnership. (Ref: Handbook Chapter B-3.)

L

LABOR AND MATERIAL PAYMENT BOND: A bond of the Contractor in which a surety guarantees to the Owner that the Contractor will pay for labor and materials used in the performance of the Contract. The claimants under the bond are defined as those having direct contracts with the Contractor or any Subcontractor. A **LABOR AND MATERIAL PAYMENT BOND** is sometimes referred to as a **PAYMENT BOND**. (Ref: AIA Document A311 and Handbook Chapter B-2.)

LAND SURVEY: See (1) **BOUNDARY SURVEY**; (2) **SURVEY**.

LATENT DEFECT: A defect in materials, equipment or completed work which reasonably careful observation could not have discovered; distinguished from a patent defect, which may be discovered by reasonable observation. See **PATENT DEFECT**.

LETTER FORM OF AGREEMENT or **LETTER AGREEMENT**: A letter stating the terms of an Agreement between addressor and addressee, usually prepared to be signed by the addressee to indicate acceptance of those terms as legally binding. (Ref: Handbook Chapter D-1.)

LETTER OF INTENT: A letter signifying an intention to enter into a formal agreement, usually setting forth the general terms of such agreement. (Ref: Handbook Chapter D-1.)

LETTING (BID): See **BID OPENING**.

LIABILITY INSURANCE: Insurance which protects the insured against liability on account of injury to the person or property of another. See also (1) **COMPLETED OPERATIONS INSURANCE**; (2) **COMPREHENSIVE GENERAL LIABILITY INSURANCE**; (3) **CONTRACTOR'S LIABILITY INSURANCE**; (4) **EMPLOYER'S LIABILITY INSURANCE**; (5) **OWNER'S LIABILITY**

INSURANCE; (6) PROFESSIONAL LIABILITY INSURANCE; (7) PROPERTY DAMAGE INSURANCE; (8) PUBLIC LIABILITY INSURANCE; (9) SPECIAL HAZARDS INSURANCE.

LICENSED ARCHITECT: See ARCHITECT.

LICENSED CONTRACTOR: A person or entity certified by governmental authority, where required by law, to engage in construction contracting.

LICENSED ENGINEER: See PROFESSIONAL ENGINEER.

LIEN: See MECHANIC'S LIEN.

LIMIT OF LIABILITY: The maximum amount which an insurance company agrees to pay in case of loss.

LIQUIDATED DAMAGES: A sum established in a Construction Contract, usually as a fixed sum per day, as the measure of damages suffered by the Owner due to failure to complete the Work within a stipulated time. See also (1) **BONUS AND PENALTY CLAUSE;** (2) **BONUS CLAUSE;** (3) **PENALTY CLAUSE.** (Ref: Handbook Chapter D-5.)

LOSS OF USE INSURANCE: Insurance protecting against financial loss during the time required to repair or replace property damaged or destroyed by an insured peril. (Ref: Handbook Chapter B-2.)

LOW BID: Bid stating the lowest bid price for performance of the Work, including selected alternates, conforming with the Bidding Documents. (Ref: AIA Document A501.)

LOWEST QUALIFIED BIDDER: See LOWEST RESPONSIBLE BIDDER.

LOWEST RESPONSIBLE BIDDER: Bidder who submits the lowest bona fide bid and is considered by the Owner and the Architect to be fully responsible and qualified to perform the Work for which the bid is submitted.

LOWEST RESPONSIVE BID: The lowest bid which is responsive to and complies with the requirements of the Bidding Documents.

LUMP SUM AGREEMENT: See STIPULATED SUM AGREEMENT.

M

MANDATORY AND CUSTOMARY BENEFITS: See BENEFITS, MANDATORY AND CUSTOMARY.

MATERIAL SUPPLIER: See SUPPLIER.

MECHANIC'S LIEN: A lien on real property created by statute in all states in favor of persons supplying labor or materials for a building or structure for the value of labor or materials supplied by them. In some jurisdictions a mechanic's lien also exists for the value of professional services. Clear title to the property cannot be obtained until the claim for the labor, materials or professional services is settled. (Ref: Handbook Chapter B-3.)

MEMORANDUM OF INSURANCE: See CERTIFICATE OF INSURANCE.

METES AND BOUNDS: The boundaries, property lines or limits of a parcel of land, defined by distances and compass directions.

MINOR CHANGES IN THE WORK: Changes of a minor nature in the Work not involving an adjustment in the Contract Sum or an extension of the Contract Time and not inconsistent with the intent of the Contract Documents, which shall be effected by written order issued by the Architect. (Ref: AIA Documents A201 and G710, and Handbook Chapter B-7.)

MODIFICATION (to the Contract Documents): (1) A written amendment to the Contract signed by both parties. (2) A Change Order. (3) A written interpretation issued by the Architect. (4) A written order for a minor change in the Work issued by the Architect. See also (1) **CHANGE ORDER;** (2) **CHANGES IN THE WORK;** (3) **MINOR CHANGES IN THE WORK.**

MODULE: (1) A repetitive dimensional or functional unit used in planning, recording or constructing buildings or other structure. (2) A distinct component forming part of an ordered system.

MORTGAGE CLAUSE/MORTGAGEE CLAUSE: A provision in a fire or other direct-damage insurance policy covering mortgaged property which states that, in the event of loss, the mortgagee shall be paid to the extent of the mortgagee's interest in the property. No violation of the policy conditions by the insured voids the policy as to the mortgagee. The clause also gives the mortgagee other rights and privileges.

MULTIPLE OF DIRECT PERSONNEL EXPENSE: A method of compensation for professional services based on Direct Personnel Expense multiplied by an agreed factor to cover indirect expenses, other direct expense and profit. See **DIRECT PERSONNEL EXPENSE.** (Ref: AIA Documents B141, B161, B171, B181 and C141 and Handbook Chapter D-1.)

MULTIPLE OF DIRECT SALARY EXPENSE: A method of compensation for professional services based on Direct Salary Expense multiplied by an agreed factor to cover the cost of contributions and benefits related to Direct Salary Expense, indirect expenses, other direct expense and profit. (Ref: AIA Documents B141, B161, B171, B181 and C141, and Handbook Chapter D-1.)

MULTIPLIER: The factor by which an Architect's Direct Personnel Expense or Direct Salary Expense is multiplied to determine compensation for professional services or designated portions thereof. (Ref: AIA Documents B141, B161, B171, B181 and C141, and Handbook Chapter D-1.)

N

NAMED INSURED: Any person, firm or corporation, or any of its members specifically designated by name as insured(s) in a policy, as distinguished from others who, although unnamed, are protected under some circumstances.

NAMED PERILS: A method of writing a contract of insurance which specifies those perils which are covered, as opposed to "All Risk" coverage which covers all perils except those specifically excluded.

NEGLIGENCE: Failure to exercise due care under the circumstances. Legal liability for the consequences of an act or omission frequently depends upon whether or not there has been negligence. See also **DUE CARE.**

NEGOTIATION PHASE: See **BIDDING OR NEGOTIATION PHASE.**

NET ASSIGNABLE AREA: See **STANDARD NET ASSIGNABLE AREA.**

NONCOLLUSION AFFIDAVIT: Notarized statement by a Bidder that the Bid was prepared without collusion of any kind.

NONCONFORMING WORK: Work that does not fulfill the requirements of the Contract Documents. (Ref: AIA Document A201.)

NOTICE TO BIDDERS: A notice contained in the Bidding Documents informing prospective bidders of the opportunity to submit bids on a Project and setting forth the procedures for doing so. See also **INSTRUCTIONS TO BIDDERS.** (Ref: AIA Document A501 and A701, and Handbook Chapter D-4.)

NOTICE TO PROCEED: Written communication issued by the Owner to the Contractor authorizing him to proceed with the Work and establishing the date of commencement of the Work. (Ref: AIA Document A201 and Handbook Chapters B-7 and D-5.)

O

OBSERVATION OF THE WORK: A function of the Architect in the Construction Phase, during visits to the site, to become generally familiar with the progress and quality of the Work and to determine in general if the Work is proceeding in accordance with the Contract Documents. See also **CONSTRUCTION PHASE-ADMINISTRATION OF THE CONSTRUCTION CONTRACT.** (Ref: AIA Documents A201, B141, B151, B161, B162, B171 and B181.)

OCCUPANCY PERMIT: See **CERTIFICATE OF OCCUPANCY.**

OCCUPATIONAL ACCIDENT: Accident occurring in the course of one's employment and caused by inherent or related hazards.

OCCURRENCE (insurance terminology): An accident or a continuous or repeated exposure to conditions which result in injury or damage, provided the injury or damage is neither expected nor intended. See **ACCIDENT.**

OCCURRENCE FORM: An insuring agreement which covers claims arising from both accidents and occurrences, as opposed to the more limited accident-only form. See also (1) **ACCIDENT;** (2) **OCCURRENCE.**

OPENING OF BIDS: See **BID OPENING.**

OPTION (CONTRACTOR'S): See **CONTRACTOR'S OPTION.**

OR EQUAL: See **APPROVED EQUAL.**

OUTLINE SPECIFICATIONS: An abbreviated listing of specification requirements normally included with schematic or design development documents.

OUT-OF-SEQUENCE SERVICES: Services performed in other than the normal or natural order of succession. (Ref: AIA Documents B141, B162, B171 and C141.)

OVERHEAD EXPENSE: See **INDIRECT EXPENSE.**

OWNER: (1) The Architect's client and party to the Owner-Architect Agreement. (2) The Owner of the Project and party to the Owner-Contractor Agreement.

OWNER-ARCHITECT AGREEMENT: Contract between Owner and Architect for professional services. (Ref: AIA Documents B141, B151, B161, B171, B181 and B727 and Handbook Chapter D-1.)

OWNER-CONTRACTOR AGREEMENT: Contract between Owner and Contractor for performance of the Work for construction of the Project or portion thereof. See also **WORK** (capital W). (Ref: AIA Documents A101, A107, A111 and A117 and Handbook Chapter D-5.)

OWNER'S INSPECTOR: A person employed by the Owner to inspect construction in the Owner's behalf. See also **CLERK OF THE WORKS.**

OWNER'S LIABILITY INSURANCE: Insurance to protect the Owner against claims arising out of the operations performed for the Owner by the Contractor and arising out of the Owner's general supervision of such operations.

OWNER'S REPRESENTATIVE: The person designated as the official representative of the Owner in connection with a Project.

P

PACKAGE DEALER: See **DESIGN-BUILD PROCESS.**

PARAGRAPH: In the AIA Documents, the first subdivision of an Article, identified by two numerals (e.g., 2.2). A paragraph may be further subdivided into sub-paragraphs (e.g., 2.2.1) and clauses (e.g., 2.2.1.1). (Ref: Handbook Chapter B-6.)

PARTIAL OCCUPANCY: Occupancy by the Owner of a portion of a Project prior to final completion. See **FINAL COMPLETION.** (Ref: Handbook Chapter B-7.)

PARTIAL PAYMENT: See **PROGRESS PAYMENT.**

PATENT DEFECT: A defect in materials, equipment or completed work which reasonably careful observation could have discovered; distinguished from a latent defect, which could not be discovered by reasonable observation. See **LATENT DEFECT.**

PAYMENT BOND: See **LABOR AND MATERIAL PAYMENT BOND.**

PAYMENT REQUEST: See **APPLICATION FOR PAYMENT.**

PENAL SUM: The amount named in a contract or bond as the penalty to be paid by a signatory thereto in the event the contractual obligations are not performed.

PENALTY AND BONUS CLAUSE: See **BONUS AND PENALTY CLAUSE.**

PENALTY CLAUSE: A provision in a contract for a charge against the Contractor for failure to complete the Work by a stipulated date. See also **LIQUIDATED DAMAGES.**

PERCENTAGE AGREEMENT: An agreement for professional services in which the compensation is based upon a percentage of the Construction Cost. (Ref: AIA Documents B141, B161, B171 and B181.)

PERCENTAGE FEE: Compensation based upon a percentage of Construction Cost. Applicable to either construction contracts or professional service agreements. See also **FEE** and **COMPENSATION.**

PERFORMANCE BOND: A bond of the Contractor in which a surety guarantees to the Owner that the Work will be performed in accordance with the Contract Documents. Except where prohibited by statute, the Performance Bond is frequently combined with the Labor and Material Payment Bond. See also **SURETY BOND.** (Ref: AIA Document A311 and Handbook Chapter B-2.)

PERMIT, BUILDING: See **BUILDING PERMIT.**

PERMIT, OCCUPANCY: See **CERTIFICATE OF OCCUPANCY.**

PERMIT, ZONING: See **ZONING PERMIT.**

PERSONAL INJURY (insurance terminology): Bodily injury, and also injury or damage to the character or reputation of a person. Personal injury insurance includes coverage for injuries or damage to others caused by specified actions of the insured such as false arrest; malicious prosecution; willful detention or imprisonment; libel, slander, defamation of character, wrongful eviction; invasion of privacy; or wrongful entry. See also **BODILY INJURY**. (Ref: Handbook Chapter B-2.)

PERSPECTIVE DRAWING: A graphic representation of the Project or part thereof as it would appear three-dimensionally.

PERT SCHEDULE: An acronym for Project Evaluation Review Technique. The Pert Schedule charts the activities and events anticipated in a work process. See also **CRITICAL PATH METHOD (CPM)**.

PLAN: A two-dimensional graphic representation of the design, location and dimensions of the Project, or parts thereof, seen in a horizontal plane viewed from above. See also **DRAWINGS**. (Ref: Handbook Chapter B-6.)

PLAN DEPOSIT: See **DEPOSIT FOR BIDDING DOCUMENTS**.

POST-CONSTRUCTION SERVICES: (1) Under traditional forms of agreement, additional services rendered after issuance of the final Certificate for Payment, or in the absence of a final Certificate for Payment, more than sixty days after the Date of Substantial Completion of the Work; or (2) under designated services forms of agreement, services necessary to assist the Owner in the use and occupancy of the facility. (Ref: AIA Documents B141, B151, B162 and B171, and Handbook Chapter D-1.)

POWER OF ATTORNEY: An instrument authorizing another to act as one's agent. See also **ATTORNEY-IN-FACT**.

PREDESIGN SERVICES: Additional services of the Architect provided prior to and preceding the customary Basic Services, including services to assist the Owner in establishing the program, financial and time requirements and limitations for the Project. See also **PROGRAMMING PHASE**. (Ref: AIA Document B161 and Handbook Chapter D-1.)

PRELIMINARY DRAWINGS: Drawings prepared during the early stages of the design of a Project. See also (1) **SCHEMATIC DESIGN PHASE**; (2) **DESIGN DEVELOPMENT PHASE**. (Ref: AIA Documents B141, B151, B162, C141 and C161.)

PRELIMINARY ESTIMATE: See **STATEMENT OF PROBABLE CONSTRUCTION COST**.

PREQUALIFICATION OF BIDDERS: The process of investigating the qualifications of prospective bidders on the basis of their experience, availability and capability for the contemplated Project and approving qualified Bidders. (Ref: AIA Documents A305 and A501, and Handbook Chapter D-4.)

PRIME CONTRACT: Contract between Owner and Contractor for construction of the Project or portion thereof.

PRIME CONTRACTOR: Any Contractor on a Project having a contract directly with the Owner.

PRIME PROFESSIONAL: Any person or entity having a contract directly with the Owner for professional services.

PRINCIPAL (in professional practice): Any person legally responsible for the activities of a professional practice.

PRINCIPAL-IN-CHARGE: The Architect or Engineer in a professional practice firm charged with the responsibility for the firm's services in connection with a given Project.

PROBABLE CONSTRUCTION COST: See **STATEMENT OF PROBABLE CONSTRUCTION COST**.

PRODUCER: Manufacturer, processor or assembler of building materials or equipment.

PRODUCT DATA: Illustrations, standard schedules, performance charts, instructions, brochures, diagrams and other information furnished by the Contractor to illustrate a material, product or system for some portion of the Work.

PRODUCTS LIABILITY INSURANCE: Insurance for liability imposed for damages caused by an occurrence arising out of goods or products manufactured, sold, handled or distributed by the insured or others trading under the insured's name. Occurrence must occur after product has been relinquished to others and away from premises of the insured. See also **COMPLETED OPERATIONS INSURANCE**.

PROFESSIONAL ADVISOR An Architect engaged by the Owner to direct a design competition for the selection of an Architect. (Ref: AIA Document J5000.)

PROFESSIONAL ENGINEER: Designation reserved, usually by law, for a person professionally qualified and duly licensed to perform engineering services such as structural, mechanical, electrical, sanitary, civil, etc. (Ref: Handbook Chapter D-2.)

PROFESSIONAL FEE: See **FEE.**

PROFESSIONAL LIABILITY INSURANCE: Insurance coverage for the insured professional's legal liability for claims for damages sustained by others allegedly as a result of negligent acts, errors, or omissions in the performance of professional services. See also **NEGLIGENCE.**

PROFESSIONAL PRACTICE: The practice of one of the environmental design professions in which services are rendered within the framework of recognized professional ethics and standards and applicable legal requirements. See **ENVIRONMENTAL DESIGN PROFESSIONS.** (Ref: AIA Document J5000.)

PROGRAM: A written statement setting forth design objectives, constraints and criteria for a Project, including space requirements and relationships, flexibility and expandability, special equipment and systems and site requirements.

PROGRAMMING PHASE: That phase of the environmental design process in which the Owner provides full information regarding requirements for the Project, including a program. See also **PREDESIGN SERVICES.** (Ref: AIA Documents B162 and D200, and Handbook Chapter D-1.)

PROGRESS PAYMENT: Partial payment made during progress of the Work on account of Work completed and/or materials suitably stored. (Ref: AIA Documents A101, A107, A111, A117, A201, B141, B151, B162, B171, B181 and C141.)

PROGRESS SCHEDULE: A diagram, graph or other pictorial or written schedule showing proposed and actual times of starting and completion of the various elements of the Work. See also (1) **CRITICAL PATH METHOD (CPM);** (2) **PERT SCHEDULE.** (Ref: AIA Document A201.)

PROJECT: (1) The total construction of which the Work performed under the Contract Documents may be the whole or a part. (2) The total furniture, furnishings and equipment and interior construction of which the Work performed under the Contract Documents may be the whole or a part. (Ref: AIA Documents A201 and A271.)

PROJECT APPLICATION FOR PAYMENT: Certified requests for payment from individual Contractors on a Construction Management Project, assembled for certification by the Architect and submittal to the Owner. See also **APPLICATION FOR PAYMENT.** (Ref: AIA Documents A101/CM, A201/CM, G722 and G723, and Handbook Chapter B-7.)

PROJECT ARCHITECT: The Architect designated by the principal-in-charge to manage the firm's services related to a given Project. See also **PROJECT MANAGER.**

PROJECT BUDGET: See **BUDGET, PROJECT.**

PROJECT CERTIFICATE FOR PAYMENT: A statement from the Architect to the Owner on a Construction Management Project confirming the amounts due individual Contractors, where multiple Contractors have separate direct agreements with the Owner. See also **CERTIFICATE FOR PAYMENT.** (Ref: AIA Documents A101/CM, A201/CM, B141/CM, G722 and G723 and Handbook Chapter B-7.)

PROJECT COST: Total cost of the Project including Construction Cost, professional compensation, land costs, furnishings and equipment, financing and other charges.

PROJECT DESIGNER: (1, Architect's office) The individual designated by the principal-in-charge to be responsible for setting the overall direction of the architectural design of a given Project. (2, Consultant's office) The individual who is responsible for the design of a specific portion of a Project, such as structural, mechanical, electrical, sanitary, civil, acoustical, food service and the like. See also **PROJECT ENGINEER.**

PROJECT ENGINEER: The Engineer, either in the Architect's office or the Consultant's office as the case may be, designated to be responsible for the design and management of specific engineering portions of a Project.

PROJECT MANAGER: A term frequently used interchangeably with Project Architect to identify the individual designated by the principal-in-charge to manage the firm's services related to a given Project. Normally these services include administrative responsibilities as well as technical responsibilities. (Ref: Handbook Chapter B-5.)

PROJECT MANUAL: The volume(s) of Document(s) prepared by the Architect for a Project which may include the bidding requirements, sample forms and Conditions of the Contract and the Specifications. (Ref: Handbook Chapter D-4 and AIA Document A511.)

PROJECT REPRESENTATIVE: The Architect's representative at the Project site who assists in the Administration of the Construction Contract. (Ref: AIA Documents B141, B162, B171, B181 and B352.)

PROJECT SITE: See **SITE**.

PROPERTY DAMAGE INSURANCE: Insurance coverage for the insured's legal liability for claims for injury to or destruction of tangible property including loss of use resulting therefrom, but usually not including coverage for injury to or destruction of property which is in the care, custody and control of the insured. See also **CARE, CUSTODY, & CONTROL.** (Ref: AIA Document A201 and Handbook Chapter B-2.)

PROPERTY INSURANCE: Coverage for loss or damage to the Work at the site caused by the perils of fire, lightning, extended coverage perils, vandalism and malicious mischief and additional perils (as otherwise provided or requested). Property insurance may be written on (1) the completed value form in which the policy is written at the start of a Project in a predetermined amount representing the insurable value of the Work (consisting of the contract sum less the cost of specified exclusions) and adjusted to the final insurable cost on completion of the Work, or (2) the reporting form in which the property values fluctuate during the policy term, requiring monthly statements showing the increase in value of Work in place over the previous month. See also (1) **ALL RISK INSURANCE;** (2) **BUILDER'S RISK INSURANCE;** (3) **EXTENDED COVERAGE INSURANCE; INSURABLE VALUE; SPECIAL HAZARDS INSURANCE.** (Ref: AIA Document A201 and Handbook Chapter B-2.)

PROPOSAL (CONTRACTOR'S): See **BID**.

PROPOSAL FORM: See **BID FORM**.

PROXIMATE CAUSE: The cause of an injury or of damages which, in natural and continuous sequence, unbroken by any legally recognized intervening cause, produces the injury, and without which the result would not have occurred. Existence of proximate cause involves both (1) causation in fact, i.e., that the wrongdoer actually produced an injury or damages, and (2) a public policy determination that the wrongdoer should be held responsible.

PUBLIC LIABILITY INSURANCE: Insurance covering liability of the insured for negligent acts resulting in bodily injury, disease or death of persons other than employees of the insured, and/or property damage. See also (1) **COMPREHENSIVE GENERAL LIABILITY INSURANCE;** (2) **CONTRACTOR'S LIABILITY INSURANCE.** (Ref: Handbook Chapter B-2.)

PUNCH LIST: See **INSPECTION LIST**.

Q

QUANTITY SURVEY: Detailed listing and quantities of all items of material and equipment necessary to construct a Project. (Ref: Handbook Chapter B-5.)

QUOTATION: A price quoted by a Contractor, Subcontractor, material supplier or vendor to furnish materials, labor or both.

R

REASONABLE CARE AND SKILL: See **DUE CARE**.

RECORD DRAWINGS: Construction drawings revised to show significant changes made during the construction process, usually based on marked-up prints, drawings and other data furnished by the Contractor to the Architect. Preferable to **AS-BUILT DRAWINGS**.

REGISTERED ARCHITECT: See **ARCHITECT**.

REIMBURSABLE EXPENSES: Amounts expended for or on account of the Project which, in accordance with the terms of the appropriate agreement, are to be reimbursed by the Owner. (Ref: AIA Documents A111, B141, B151, B161, B171, B181, and C141.)

REJECTION OF WORK (by the Architect): The act of rejecting Work which is defective or does not conform to the requirements of the Contract Documents. (Ref: AIA Document A201 and Handbook Chapter D-3.)

RELEASE OF LIEN: Instrument executed by a person or entity supplying labor, materials or professional services on a Project which releases that person's or entity's mechanic's lien against the Project property. See also **MECHANIC'S LIEN** and **WAIVER OF LIEN**. (Ref: AIA Document G706A and Handbook Chapter B-7.)

REMODELING: See **ALTERATIONS**.

REPORTING FORM PROPERTY INSURANCE: See **PROPERTY INSURANCE**.

REQUEST FOR A CHANGE: See **BULLETIN**.

RENDERING: A drawing of a Project or portion thereof with an artistic delineation of materials, shades and shadows.

REQUEST FOR PAYMENT: See **APPLICATION FOR PAYMENT**.

RESIDENT ENGINEER: An engineer employed by the Owner to represent the Owner's interests at the Project site during the Construction Phase; term frequently used on Projects in which a governmental agency is involved. See also **OWNER'S INSPECTOR** and **CLERK OF THE WORKS**.

RESIDENT INSPECTOR: See (1) **OWNER'S INSPECTOR**; (2) **RESIDENT ENGINEER**. See also **PROJECT REPRESENTATIVE**.

RESPONSIBLE BIDDER: See **LOWEST RESPONSIBLE BIDDER**.

RESTRICTED LIST OF BIDDERS: See **INVITED BIDDERS**.

RETAINAGE: A sum withheld from progress payments to the Contractor in accordance with the terms of the Owner-Contractor Agreement. (Ref: AIA Documents A101, A107, A111, A117, A511 and A201, and Handbook Chapter B-7.)

RETAINED PERCENTAGE: See **RETAINAGE**.

S

SAMPLES: Physical examples which illustrate materials, equipment or workmanship and establish standards by which the Work will be judged. (Ref: AIA Document A201.)

SCHEDULE: (1, drawings) A supplemental listing, usually in chart form, of a Project system, subsystem or portion thereof. See also **DRAWINGS**. (2, specifications) A detailed written listing included in the specifications. See **PROGRESS SCHEDULE**.

SCHEDULE OF VALUES: A statement furnished by the Contractor to the Architect reflecting the portions of the Contract Sum allocated to the various portions of the Work and used as the basis for reviewing the Contractor's Applications for Payment. Preferable to **CONTRACTOR'S BREAKDOWN**. (Ref: AIA Documents A201, G702, G703 and Handbook Chapter B-7.)

SCHEMATIC DESIGN DOCUMENTS: Drawings and other documents illustrating the scale and relationship of Project components. (Ref: B141 and B162.)

SCHEMATIC DESIGN PHASE: The Phase of the Architect's Services in which the Architect consults with the Owner to ascertain the requirements of the Project and prepares Schematic Design studies consisting of drawings and other documents illustrating the scale and relationship of the Project components for approval by the Owner. The Architect also submits to the Owner a Statement of Probable Construction Cost based on current area, volume or other unit costs. (Ref: AIA Documents B141, B151, B162, B171 and D200, and Handbook Chapters B-4 and D-1.)

SEAL: (1) An embossing device, stamp or other device used by a design professional on Drawings and Specifications as evidence of registration in the state where the Work is to be performed. (2) A device formerly consisting of an impression upon wax or paper, or a wafer, which is used in the execution of a formal legal document such as a deed or contract. The statute of limitations applicable to a contract under seal may be longer than for a contract not under seal. (Ref: Handbook Chapter B-3.)

SECTION: (1, drawing) A drawing of a surface revealed by an imaginary plane cut through the Project, or portion thereof, in such a manner as to show the composition of the surface as it would appear if the part intervening between the cut plane and the eye of the observer were removed. See also **DRAWINGS**. (2, of Specifications) A subdivision of a Division of the Specifications which covers a unit of Work. (Ref: Handbook Chapter B-6.)

SELECTED BIDDER: The bidder selected by the Owner for discussions relative to the possible award of a construction contract.

SELECTED LIST OF BIDDERS: See INVITED BIDDERS.

SEPARATE CONTRACT: One of several prime contracts for construction of the Project.

SEPARATE CONTRACTOR: A Contractor on a Project having a separate contract with the Owner.

SHOP DRAWINGS: Drawings, diagrams, schedules and other data specially prepared for the Work by the Contractor or any Subcontractor, manufacturer, supplier or distributor to illustrate some portion of the Work. (Ref: AIA Document A201 and Handbook Chapter B-6.)

SINGLE CONTRACT: Contract for construction of the Project under which a single prime Contractor is responsible for all of the Work.

SITE: Geographical location of the Project, usually defined by legal boundary lines.

SITE ANALYSIS SERVICES (of the Architect): Those services described in the schedule of designated services necessary to establish site related limitations and requirements for the Project. (Ref: AIA Documents B161 and B162.)

SOIL SURVEY: See SUBSURFACE INVESTIGATION.

SPECIAL CONDITIONS: A section of the Conditions of the Contract, other than General Conditions and Supplementary Conditions, which may be prepared to describe conditions unique to a particular Project. See also CONDITIONS OF THE CONTRACT.

SPECIAL HAZARDS INSURANCE: Insurance coverage for damage caused by additional perils or risks to be included in the Property Insurance (at the request of the Contractor or at the option of the Owner). Examples often included are sprinkler leakage, collapse, water damage, and coverage for materials in transit to the site or stored off the site. See PROPERTY INSURANCE. (Ref: AIA Document A201 and Handbook Chapter B-2.)

SPECIFICATIONS: A part of the Contract Documents contained in the Project Manual consisting of written requirements for materials, equipment, construction systems, standards and workmanship. Under the Uniform Construction Index, the Specifications comprise sixteen Divisions. (Ref: Handbook Chapter B-6.)

SPECULATIVE BUILDER: One who develops and constructs building projects for subsequent sale or lease.

STANDARD NET ASSIGNABLE AREA: That portion of the area of a Project which is available for assignment or rental to an occupant, including every type of space usable by the occupant, computed in accordance with AIA Document D101. (Ref: AIA Document D101.)

STATEMENTS OF ETHICAL PRINCIPLES: Statements of ethical principles promulgated by professional societies to guide their members in the conduct of professional practice. (Ref: AIA Document 6J400.)

STATEMENT OF PROBABLE CONSTRUCTION COST: Cost forecasts prepared by the Architect during the Schematic Design, Design Development and Construction Documents Phases of Basic Services for the guidance of the Owner. (Ref: AIA Documents B141, B151, B162, B171 and C141 and Handbook Chapter B-5.)

STATUTE OF LIMITATIONS: A statute specifying the period of time within which legal action must be brought for alleged damage or injury, or other legal relief. The lengths of the periods vary from state to state and depend upon the type of legal action. Ordinarily, the period commences with the occurrence of the damage or injury, or discovery of the act resulting in the alleged damage or injury. In construction industry cases, many jurisdictions define the period as commencing with completion of the Work or services performed in connection therewith.

STATUTORY BOND: A bond, the form or content of which is prescribed by statute. (Ref: Handbook Chapter B-2.)

STEAM BOILER AND MACHINERY INSURANCE: See BOILER AND MACHINERY INSURANCE.

STIPULATED SUM AGREEMENT: Contract in which a specific amount is set forth as the total payment for performance of the Contract. (Ref: AIA Documents A101, A107, A171 and A177.)

STUDY: Preliminary sketch or drawing to facilitate the development of a design.

SUB-BIDDER: A person or entity who submits a bid to a Bidder for materials or labor for a portion of the Work.

SUBCONTRACT: Agreement between a prime Contractor and a Subcontractor for a portion of the Work at the site. (Ref: AIA Document A401 and Handbook Chapter D-5.)

SUBCONTRACTOR: A person or entity who has a direct contract with the Contractor to perform any of the Work at the site. See also **SUPPLIER, VENDOR.** (Ref: AIA Document A201 and A401, and Handbook Chapter D-5.)

SUBHEADING: A subdivision of a **HEADING** used in the Filing System.

SUBPARAGRAPH: In the AIA Documents, the first subdivision of a Paragraph, identified by three numerals (e.g., 2.2.2). A Subparagraph may be subdivided into clauses.

SUBROGATION: The substitution of one person or entity for another with respect to legal rights such as a right of recovery. Subrogation occurs when a third person such as an insurance company, has paid a debt of another or claim against another and succeeds to all legal rights which the debtor or person against whom the claim was asserted may have against other persons.

SUBSTANTIAL COMPLETION: See **DATE OF SUBSTANTIAL COMPLETION.**

SUBSTITUTION: A material, product or item of equipment offered in lieu of that specified.

SUB-SUBCONTRACTOR: A person or entity who has a direct or indirect Contract with a Subcontractor to perform any of the Work at the site.

SUBSURFACE INVESTIGATION (sometimes called Geotechnical Investigation): The soil boring and sampling program, together with the associated laboratory tests, necessary to establish subsurface profiles and the relative strengths, compressibility and other characteristics of the various strata encountered within depths likely to have an influence on the design of the Project. Preferable to **SOIL SURVEY.** (Ref: AIA Document G602.)

SUCCESSFUL BIDDER: The bidder chosen by the Owner for the award of a construction contract. See also **SELECTED BIDDER.** (Ref: AIA Document A501.)

SUPERINTENDENT: Contractor's representative at the site who is responsible for continuous field supervision, coordination, completion of the Work and, unless another person is designated in writing by the Contractor to the Owner and the Architect, for the prevention of accidents. (Ref: AIA Document A201.)

SUPERVISION: Direction of the Work by Contractor's personnel. Supervision is neither a duty nor a responsibility of the Architect as part of professional services.

SUPPLEMENTAL AUTHORIZATION (Professional Services): Written agreement authorizing a modification to a professional services agreement. (Ref: AIA Document G604.)

SUPPLEMENTAL CONDITIONS: See **SUPPLEMENTARY CONDITIONS.**

SUPPLEMENTAL SERVICES (of the Architect): Those services described in the schedule of Designated Services which are in addition to the generally sequential services (from Predesign through Postconstruction) of the Architect, including such items of service as renderings, value analyses, energy studies, project promotion, expert testimony and the like. (Ref: AIA Documents B161 and B162.)

SUPPLEMENTARY CONDITIONS: A part of the Contract Documents which supplements and may also modify, change, add to or delete from provisions of the General Conditions. See also **CONDITIONS OF THE CONTRACT.** Preferable to **SUPPLEMENTAL CONDITIONS.** (Ref: Handbook Chapter D-3.)

SUPPLIER: A person or entity who supplies materials or equipment for the Work, including that fabricated to a special design, but who does not perform labor at the site. See also **VENDOR.**

SURETY: A person or entity who promises in writing to make good the debt or default of another. (Ref: Handbook Chapter B-2.)

SURETY BOND: A legal instrument under which one party agrees to answer to another party for the debt, default or failure to perform of a third party. (Ref: Handbook Chapter B-2.)

SURVEY: (1) Boundary, topographic and/or utility mapping of a site. (2) Measuring an existing building. (3) Analyzing a building for use of space. (4) Determining Owner's requirements for a Project. (5) Investigating and reporting of required data for a Project.

SYSTEMS (a process): Combining prefabricated assemblies, components and parts into single integrated units utilizing industrialized production, assembly and methods.

T

TERMINATION EXPENSES (Professional Services): Expenses directly attributable to the termination of a professional services agreement, including an amount allowing for compensation earned to the time of termination. (Ref: AIA Document B141, B151, B161, B171, B181, C141 and C161.)

TIME (as the essence of a construction contract): Time limits or periods stated in the Contract. A provision in a construction contract that "time is of the essence of the contract" signifies that the parties consider punctual performance within the time limits or periods in the Contract to be a vital part of the performance, and failure to perform on time is a breach for which the injured party is entitled to damages in the amount of loss sustained.

TIME OF COMPLETION: Date established in the Contract, by calendar date or by number of days, for Substantial Completion of the Work. See also (1) **DATE OF SUBSTANTIAL COMPLETION;** (2) **CONTRACT TIME.**

TIMELY COMPLETION: Completion of the Work or designated portion thereof on or before the date required.

TOPOGRAPHIC SURVEY: The configuration of a surface including its relief and the locations of its natural and man-made features, usually recorded on a drawing showing surface variations by means of contour lines indicating height above or below a fixed datum.

TRADE (CRAFT): (1) Occupation requiring manual skill. (2) Members of a trade organized into a collective body.

TRADE DISCOUNT: The difference between the seller's list price and the purchaser's actual cost, excluding discounts for prompt payment.

U

UMBRELLA LIABILITY INSURANCE: Insurance providing excess liability coverage over existing liability policies such as Employer's Liability, General Liability or Automobile Liability, and providing direct coverage for many losses uninsured under the existing policies after a specified deductible is exceeded. See also **EXCESS LIABILITY INSURANCE.** (Ref: Handbook Chapter B-2.)

UNIFORM CONSTRUCTION INDEX: A published system for coordination of Specification sections, filing of technical data and product literature, and construction cost accounting organized into sixteen Divisions.

UNIT PRICE: Amount stated in the Bid as a price per unit of measurement for materials or services as described in the Bidding Documents or in the proposed Contract Documents.

UPSET PRICE: See **GUARANTEED MAXIMUM COST.**

UTILITY SURVEY: A survey showing existing site utilities.

V

VANDALISM AND MALICIOUS MISCHIEF INSURANCE: Insurance against loss or damage to the insured's property caused by willful and malicious damage or destruction.

VENDOR: A person or entity who furnishes materials or equipment not fabricated to a special design for the Work. See also **SUPPLIER.**

VOLUME METHOD (of estimating cost): Method of estimating Probable Construction Cost by multiplying the architectural volume by an estimated current cost per unit of volume. See also **ARCHITECTURAL VOLUME OF BUILDINGS.** See also **ARCHITECTURAL AREA OF BUILDINGS** and **AREA METHOD.** (Ref: AIA Document D101 and Handbook Chapter B-5.)

W

WAIVER OF LIEN: An instrument by which a person or organization who has or may have a right of mechanic's lien against the property of another relinquishes such right. See also (1) **MECHANIC'S LIEN;** (2) **RELEASE OF LIEN.**

WARRANTY: Legally enforceable assurance of quality or performance of a product or Work, or of the duration of satisfactory performance. **WARRANTY, GUARANTEE** and **GUARANTY** are substantially identical in meaning; nevertheless, confusion frequently arises from supposed distinctions attributed to **GUARANTEE** (or **GUARANTY**) being exclusively indicative of duration of satisfactory performance or of a legally enforceable assurance furnished by a manufacturer or other third party. The Uniform Commercial Code provisions on Sales (effective in all states except Louisiana) use **WARRAN-TY** but recognize the continuation of the use of **GUAR-ANTEE** and **GUARANTY**.

WORK (capital "W"): As used in AIA Documents, the completed construction required by the Contract Documents, including all labor necessary to produce such construction, and all materials and equipment incorporated or to be incorporated in such construction. (Ref: AIA Document A201, Subparagraph 4.4.1.) The word "work" as contrasted with capitalized "Work" is used in its ordinary sense.

WORKERS' COMPENSATION INSURANCE: Insurance covering the liability of an employer to employees for compensation and other benefits required by workers' compensation laws with respect to injury, sickness, disease or death arising from their employment. Also still known in some jurisdictions as workmen's compensation insurance. (Ref: AIA Document A201 and Handbook Chapter B-2.)

WORKING DRAWINGS: See **DRAWINGS**.

X

XCU (insurance terminology): Letters which refer to exclusions from coverage for property damage liability arising out of (1) explosion or blasting, (2) collapse of or structural damage to any building or structure, and (3) underground damage caused by and occurring during the use of mechanical equipment. (Ref: Handbook Chapter B-2.)

Z

ZONING PERMIT: A permit issued by appropriate governmental authority authorizing land to be used for a specific purpose.

BIBLIOGRAPHY

Briggs, Martin Shaw.
Everyman's Concise Encyclopedia of Architecture.
London: J. M. Dent; New York: Dutton, 1960.

Brooks, Hugh.
*Illustrated Encyclopedic Dictionary of Building and
Construction Terms.* Englewood Cliffs, N.J.: Prentice-
Hall, 1976.

Building Materials Merchandiser.
. . . Cyclopedia of Building Terms. . . . Chicago: n.p.,
1963.

Burke, Arthur Edward; Dalzell, J. Ralph; and Townsend,
Gilbert.
Architectural and Building Trades Dictionary.
Chicago: American Technical Society, 1950.

Cagnacci-Schwicker, Angelo.
International Dictionary of Building Construction.
Milan: Ulrico Hoepli Editore; distributed by Scholium
International, Flushing, New York, 1972.

Cowan, Henry J.
Dictionary of Architectural Science. New York: John
Wiley & Sons, 1973.

Del Vecchio, Alfred.
Dictionary of Mechanical Engineering. New York: Phil-
osophical Library, 1961.

Guedes, Pedro, ed.
Encyclopedia of Architectural Technology. New York:
McGraw Hill, 1979.

Harris, Cyril M.
Dictionary of Architecture and Construction. New
York: McGraw-Hill, 1975.

Hunt, William Dudley.
Encyclopedia of American Architecture. New York:
McGraw-Hill, 1980.

Kay, N. W., ed.
*The Modern Building Encyclopedia: An Authoritative
Reference to All Aspects of the Building and Allied
Trades.* London: Oldhams Press, 1955.

Lipowsky, Benjamin, and Bersten, Murray.
*A Picture Dictionary and Guide to Building and Con-
struction Terms.* New York: Arco Pub. Co., 1960.

Moskowitz, Harvey S., and Lindbloom, Carl G.
The Illustrated Book of Development Definitions.
Piscataway, N.J.: Center for Urban Policy Research,
Rutgers University, 1981.

National Association of Women in Construction, Phoenix
Chapter.
*Construction Dictionary: Construction Terms and
Tables and an Encyclopedia of Construction.* Phoenix,
Ariz.: 1973.

Pevsner, Nikolaus; Fleming, John; and Honour, Hugh.
A Dictionary of Architecture. rev. and enl. Woodstock,
N.Y.: The Overlook Press, 1976.

Putnam, R. E., and Carlson, G. E.
Architectural and Building Trades Dictionary. Chicago: American Technical Society, 1974.

Saylor, Henry Hodgman.
Dictionary of Architecture. New York: John Wiley &
Sons, 1952.

Scott, John S.
A Dictionary of Building. Baltimore: Penguin Books,
1964.

Siegele, Herman Hugo.
*Building Trades Dictionary; a Book Written in Simple
Language, Defining Words, Phrases and Expressions
Pertaining to the Building Trades.* Chicago: E. J.
Drake & Co., 1946.

Stein, J. Stewart.
*Construction Glossary: An Encyclopedic Reference
and Manual.* New York: John Wiley & Sons, 1980.

Sturgis, Russell.
*A Dictionary of Architecture and Buildings, Biographi-
cal, Historical, and Descriptive.* New York: The Macmillan Co.; London: Macmillan & Co. Ltd., 1901.

Van Mansum, C. J., comp.
*Elsevier's Dictionary of Building Construction, in Four
Languages, English/American, French, Dutch and
German.* Amsterdam, New York: Elsevier Pub. Co.,
1959.

Waugh, Herbert R., and Burbank, Nelson L.
Handbook of Building Trades and Definitions. New
York: Simmons-Boardman Pub. Corp., 1954.

White, Norval.
The Architecture Book. New York: Alfred A. Knopf,
1976.

Zboinski, A., and Tyszynski, L., eds.
*Dictionary of Architecture and Building Trades in Four
Languages: English, German, Polish, Russian.* Oxford,
New York: Pergamon Press; distributed in the Western
Hemisphere by MacMillan, New York, 1963.

Appendix B

DOCUMENTS SYNOPSES

THE AMERICAN INSTITUTE OF ARCHITECTS

THE AMERICAN INSTITUTE OF ARCHITECTS

These synopses of AIA Documents have been created by the AIA Documents Committee to provide AIA Document users with a quick reference for determining the specific applications of each AIA Document. They will also be of use to those unfamiliar with AIA Documents by providing an overview of the types of agreements covered by AIA Documents.

The synopses are listed according to series: A-Series—Owner-Contractor Agreements, B-Series—Owner-Architect Agreements, C-Series—Architect-Consultant Agreements, D-Series—Architect-Industry Agreements, G-Series—Contract Administration Forms.

While these synopses will aid users in selecting the most suitable document for a given agreement, the *Documents Synopses* should not be used as the sole basis for selection. Careful examination of the documents themselves, as well as consultation with legal counsel are advised to ensure use of the most suitable documents.

APPENDIX $\mathbb{B}$ • DOCUMENTS SYNOPSES

A-SERIES

DOCUMENTS RELATING TO THE AGREEMENT BETWEEN THE OWNER AND THE CONTRACTOR.

AIA DOCUMENT A101, OWNER-CONTRACTOR AGREEMENT FORM–STIPULATED SUM

This is a standard form of agreement between owner and contractor, for use where the basis of payment is a stipulated sum (fixed price). The document has been prepared for use with AIA Document A201, *General Conditions of the Contract for Construction,* providing an integrated pair of documents. This pair of documents is suitable for most projects; however, for projects of limited scope, use of AIA Document A107 should be considered.

AIA DOCUMENT A101/CM, OWNER-CONTRACTOR AGREEMENT FORM–STIPULATED SUM –CONSTRUCTION MANAGEMENT EDITION

This is a standard form of agreement between owner and contractor, for use where the basis of payment is a stipulated sum (fixed price), on projects where there is a construction manager. The document has been prepared for use with AIA Document A201/CM, *General Conditions of the Contract for Construction, Construction Management Edition.* It is suitable for any arrangement between the owner and the contractor on a project with a construction manager where the construction cost has been determined in advance either by bidding or by negotiation.

AIA DOCUMENT A107, OWNER-CONTRACTOR AGREEMENT FORM–STIPULATED SUM–FOR CONSTRUCTION PROJECTS OF LIMITED SCOPE

This is an abbreviated form of agreement between owner and contractor, for use where the basis of payment is a stipulated sum (fixed price) for construction projects of limited scope not requiring the complexity and length of the combination of AIA Documents A101 and A201; especially where such complexity and length might adversely affect the bidding or negotiations of contractors who are not accustomed to dealing with those documents. The document contains abbreviated General Conditions based on AIA Document A201. The document is suitable for any arrangement between the owner and the contractor where the construction cost has been determined in advance either by bidding or by negotiation.

AIA DOCUMENT A111, OWNER-CONTRACTOR AGREEMENT FORM–COST OF THE WORK PLUS A FEE

This is a standard form of agreement between owner and contractor, for use where the basis of payment to the contractor is the cost of the work plus a fee, which may be a stipulated amount or a percentage of the construction cost. A guaranteed maximum construction cost may be designated, with provisions, if any, for distribution of any savings below the guaranteed maximum cost. The document has been prepared for use with AIA Document A201, *General Conditions of the Contract for Construction,* providing an integrated pair of documents. This pair of documents is suitable for most projects; however, for projects of limited scope, use of AIA Document A117 should be considered.

AIA DOCUMENT A117, OWNER-CONTRACTOR AGREEMENT FORM–COST OF THE WORK PLUS A FEE–FOR CONSTRUCTION PROJECTS OF LIMITED SCOPE

This is an abbreviated form of agreement between owner and contractor, for use where the basis of payment to the contractor is the cost of the work plus a fee, for construction projects of limited scope which do not require the complexity and length of the combination of AIA Documents A111 and A201. The document contains abbreviated General Conditions based on AIA Document A201. A guaranteed maximum construction cost may be designated, with provisions, if any, for distribution of any savings below the guaranteed maximum cost.

AIA DOCUMENT A171, OWNER-CONTRACTOR AGREEMENT FORM–STIPULATED SUM–FOR FURNITURE, FURNISHINGS AND EQUIPMENT

This is a standard form of agreement between owner and contractor for furniture, furnishings and equipment where the basis of payment is a stipulated sum (fixed price). The document has been prepared for use with AIA Document A271, *General Conditions of the Contract for Furniture, Furnishings and Equipment.* It is suitable for any arrangement between the owner and the contractor where the cost of furniture, furnishings and equipment has been determined in advance either by bidding or by negotiation.

AIA DOCUMENT A177, ABBREVIATED OWNER-CONTRACTOR AGREEMENT FORM–STIPULATED SUM–FOR FURNITURE, FURNISHINGS AND EQUIPMENT

This is an abbreviated form of agreement between owner and contractor for furniture, furnishings and equipment where the basis of payment is a stipulated sum (fixed price) for projects whose scope does not require the complexity and length of the combination of AIA Documents A171 and A271; especially where such complexity and length might adversely affect the bidding of negotiations of contractors who are not accustomed to dealing with these documents. The document contains abbreviated General Conditions based on AIA Document A271. The document is suitable for any arrangement between the owner and contractor where the cost of furniture, furnishings and equipment has been determined in advance either by bidding or by negotiation.

AIA DOCUMENT A201, GENERAL CONDITIONS OF THE CONTRACT FOR CONSTRUCTION

The *General Conditions* are a part of the contract for construction and set forth rights, responsibilities and relationships of the parties involved. Since conditions vary by locality and project, supplementary conditions are usually required to amend or supplement portions of the *General Conditions* as required by the individual project.

While not a party to the owner-contractor agreement and the general conditions thereof, the architect does participate in the preparation of the contract documents and performs certain of the duties and responsibilities assigned thereunder.

AIA DOCUMENT A201/CM, GENERAL CONDITIONS OF THE CONTRACT FOR CONSTRUCTION–CONSTRUCTION MANAGEMENT EDITION

A201/CM is an adaptation of AIA Document A201 for construction management projects where the services, duties and responsibilities of the construction manager are as described in AIA Document B801, *Standard Form of Agreement Between Owner and Construction Manager.* A major difference between A201 and A201/CM occurs in Article 2. Article 2 of A201/CM is entitled Administration Of The Contract and deals with the duties and responsibilities of both the architect and the construction manager. Another major difference is the use of multiple direct contracts with no general contractor.

AIA DOCUMENT A201/SC, FEDERAL SUPPLEMENTARY CONDITIONS OF THE CONTRACT FOR CONSTRUCTION

A201/SC is published and distributed only with A201, and the documents are intended for joint use on certain federally assisted construction projects. For such projects, A201/SC adapts A201 by providing (1) necessary modifications of the General Conditions, (2) additional conditions, and (3) insurance requirements for federally assisted construction projects.

AIA DOCUMENT A271, GENERAL CONDITIONS OF THE CONTRACT FOR FURNITURE, FURNISHINGS AND EQUIPMENT

When the contract scope is limited to furniture, furnishings and equipment, A271 is intended to be used in a manner similar to that in which A201 is used for construction projects. The document was developed jointly by the American Institute of Architects (AIA) and the American Society of Interior Designers (ASID). Because the Uniform Commercial Code (UCC) has been adopted in virtually every jurisdiction, A271 has been drafted to recognize the commercial standards set forth in Article 2 of the UCC, and it uses certain standard UCC terminology.

AIA DOCUMENT A305, CONTRACTOR'S QUALIFICATION STATEMENT

An owner about to request bids or to award a contract for a construction project needs a vehicle for verifying the background, history, references and financial stability of any contractor being considered. The construction time frame, the contractor's performance, history and previous similar experience, as well as financial capability are important factors for an owner to consider. This form provides a sworn, notarized statement with appropriate attachments to elaborate on the important facets of the contractor's qualifications.

AIA DOCUMENT A310, BID BOND

This simple one-page form was drafted with input from the major surety companies as to its legality and acceptability. A bid bond establishes the maximum penal amount that may be due the owner if the selected bidder fails to execute the contract and provide any required bonds.

AIA DOCUMENT A311, PERFORMANCE BOND/ LABOR AND MATERIAL PAYMENT BOND

This two-part bond form, when properly executed, guarantees the funds, up to the penal sum, to complete the contract, in the event some unforeseen situation prevents the original contractor and subcontractors from finishing the work.

The *Performance Bond* allows the surety, in the event of the contractor's default, to assume the contract obligations and "perform" the contractor's function, obtaining a bid or bids to complete the work.

Should the contractor fail to make proper payments, the *Labor and Material Payment Bond* guarantees funds for those subcontractors and others whose labor and materials are required for complete performance of the contract.

AIA DOCUMENT A311/CM, PERFORMANCE BOND/ LABOR AND MATERIAL PAYMENT BOND– CONSTRUCTION MANAGEMENT EDITION

This document serves the same purpose for construction management projects as the A311 normally serves. However, it has been modified to take into account the many separate contracts involved, each with a date of substantial completion that may be earlier than the ultimate date of substantial completion of the project.

AIA DOCUMENT A401, STANDARD FORM OF AGREEMENT BETWEEN CONTRACTOR AND SUBCONTRACTOR

This document establishes the contractual relationship between prime contractor and subcontractor. It spells out the responsibilies of both parties and lists their respective obligations as enumerated in the *General Conditions,* AIA Document A201. The appropriate sections of A201 are included as part of the document. Blank spaces are provided where the parties can supplement the details of their agreement for each project.

AIA DOCUMENT A501, RECOMMENDED GUIDE FOR COMPETITIVE BIDDING PROCEDURES AND CONTRACT AWARDS FOR BUILDING CONSTRUCTION

This guide is intended to establish desirable objectives in the bidding procedure and the award of contracts. The *Guide* is for use when competitive lump sum bids are requested in connection with building and related construction, and is a joint publication of the AIA and the Associated General Contractors of America (AGC).

AIA DOCUMENT A511, GUIDE FOR SUPPLEMENTARY CONDITIONS

AIA Document A201, the *General Conditions,* is the foundation document supporting the legal framework for the construction contract. Though extremely important, it is obvious that as a standardized document A201 cannot cover all the requirements which must be included for purposes of bidding or construction.

This guide points out the kinds of additional information most frequently required to cover local situations and variations in project requirements. Even though it suggests standardized language, it is not meant to be a standardized form of supplementary conditions. Rather, it is intended to be an aid to the practitioner in preparing supplementary conditions.

The two-color printing and two-column text makes the *Guide* easy to use and simplifies the analysis of general conditions requirements as they apply to each individual project's documentation.

AIA DOCUMENT A511/CM, GUIDE FOR SUPPLEMENTARY CONDITIONS–CONSTRUCTION MANAGEMENT EDITION

A511/CM is the guide for supplementary conditions to

be used in place of A511, when working on construction management projects. This guide generally follows the format and purpose of A511. However, important distinctions are made with respect to many aspects of a construction management project.

AIA DOCUMENT A512, ADDITIONS TO THE GUIDE FOR SUPPLEMENTARY CONDITIONS

This document is used primarily to incorporate important recent developments in construction-related law and practices into the AIA Documents occurring since the issuance of the latest editions of either A201 or A511. Thus, A512 may be revised on a shorter cycle than other AIA Documents, depending on the frequency and extent of changes in the construction industry. The document collects these changes cumulatively, and where appropriate, its provisions will be incorporated into new editions of the other AIA Documents.

AIA DOCUMENT A521, UNIFORM LOCATION OF SUBJECT MATTER

This document recognizes that there are widely varying approaches to the question of where in the contract documents a particular matter should properly be covered. The practice of many architects of addressing the same subject matter in more than one location has caused confusion and unanticipated legal problems when the exact language is not repeated each time. This tabulation is intended to guide the user in determining the proper location of information in those documents customarily used on a construction project.

The listing was not created for the exclusive use of design professionals, but also for owners, attorneys, contractors, subcontractors, lenders, sureties and others who work with construction documents.

AIA DOCUMENT A571, GUIDE FOR INTERIORS SUPPLEMENTARY CONDITIONS

Like A511 and A511/CM, AIA Document A571 is intended to aid practitioners in preparing supplementary conditions.

AIA Document A571 describes the additional information required to cover local variations in project requirements for interiors projects where A271, *General Conditions of the Contract for Furniture, Furnishings and Equipment,* is used.

AIA DOCUMENT A701, INSTRUCTIONS TO BIDDERS

This document provides a base which other documents and project requirements build upon. It is complementary to the AIA *General Conditions;* it is meant for general usage and anticipates some additions, modifications and other provisions. The usual, rather than specific, project provisions for instructions to bidders are included.

AIA DOCUMENT A771, INSTRUCTIONS TO INTERIORS BIDDERS

This document is designed for use on projects dealing with furniture, furnishings and equipment. It parallels the typical *Instructions to Bidders,* A701, with minor changes necessary to maintain consistency of language and references.

B-SERIES

DOCUMENTS RELATING TO THE AGREEMENT BETWEEN THE OWNER AND THE ARCHITECT FOR PROFESSIONAL SERVICES.

AIA DOCUMENT B141, STANDARD FORM OF AGREEMENT BETWEEN OWNER AND ARCHITECT

This is a standard form of agreement between owner and architect, for use where services are based on the five traditional phases. The document has been prepared for use when AIA Document A201, *General Conditions of the Contract for Construction,* is used in the contract between the owner and the contractor. It sets forth the duties and responsibilities of the architect and the owner in each phase of the project.

AIA DOCUMENT B141/CM, STANDARD FORM OF AGREEMENT BETWEEN OWNER AND ARCHITECT– CONSTRUCTION MANAGEMENT EDITION

This is a standard form of agreement between owner and architect, designed to be used in place of B141 on projects for which construction management services are to be provided, consistent with AIA Document B801, *Owner-Construction Manager Agreement.*

Those articles in B141/CM which do not specifically relate to the interrelationship of the construction manager and architect, are generally identical to those in B141.

AIA DOCUMENT B151, ABBREVIATED OWNER-ARCHITECT AGREEMENT

This is an abbreviated owner-architect agreement for use on projects of limited scope where a concise, readable contract is needed but the services and detail of the B141, *Owner-Architect Agreement,* may not be appropriate. Compared to B141, in B151 design services are provided in a single design phase, and there are no printed provisions for additional services or additional project representation. B151 should be used in lieu of oral or letter forms of agreement.

AIA DOCUMENT B161, STANDARD FORM OF AGREEMENT BETWEEN OWNER AND ARCHITECT FOR DESIGNATED SERVICES

This standard form of agreement between owner and architect for designated services is intended to be used in conjunction with AIA Document B162, *Scope of Designated Services.* These documents are designed to work together in describing the terms and conditions of the agreement, the amounts of compensation (B161) and the responsibilities and services to be undertaken by the owner and architect (B162). The separation of B161 and B162 provides for the flexibility of using B162, *Scope of Designated Services,* with other agreement forms. B161 may be used as the terms and conditions with other forms of scope of services statements. However, neither document may be used alone.

B161 provides a description of the architect's construction phase services which is coordinated with AIA Document A201, *General Conditions of the Contract for Construction.*

AIA DOCUMENT B162, SCOPE OF DESIGNATED SERVICES

The *Scope of Designated Services* is intended to be used in conjunction with AIA Document B161, *Owner-Architect Agreement for Designated Services.* These documents are designed to work together in describing the terms and conditions of the agreement, the amounts of compensation (B161) and the responsibilities and services to be undertaken by the owner and architect (B162). The separation of B161 and B162 provides for the flexibility of using B162, *Scope of Designated Services,* with other agreement forms. B161 may be used as the terms and conditions with other forms of scope of services statements. However, neither document may be used alone.

B162 provides for designated services to be performed by both the owner and the architect. Nine phases of services are listed from pre-design and site analysis through the traditional five phases to post-construction and supplemental services. Within the nine phases, over 125 different services are listed and more may be added at the parties' discretion. Any or all may be designated as appropriate to the project.

AIA DOCUMENT B171, STANDARD FORM OF AGREEMENT FOR INTERIOR DESIGN SERVICES

This is a standard form of agreement for interior design services, used as the basis for an independent undertaking by the architect.

When B171 is used, AIA Document A271, *General Conditions of the Contract for Furniture, Furnishings and Equipment,* should be used as a part of the contract for procurement and installation of these items.

AIA DOCUMENT B177, ABBREVIATED FORM OF AGREEMENT FOR INTERIOR DESIGN SERVICES

This is an abbreviated agreement designed for projects of limited scope. It may be used as the prime agreement with a building owner or tenant or other client, or it may be used as a consulting agreement when different parties are responsible for architectural and interior design.

AIA DOCUMENT B181, STANDARD FORM OF AGREEMENT BETWEEN OWNER AND ARCHITECT FOR HOUSING SERVICES WITH COST ESTIMATING SERVICES PROVIDED BY OWNER

The *Standard Form of Agreement Between Owner and Architect for Housing Services with Cost Estimating Services Provided by Owner* is intended for use on single and multifamily dwelling projects, including those for government agencies, and is essentially a modified version of AIA Document B151, *Abbreviated Owner-Architect Agreement.*

This document has been accepted by the U.S. Department of HUD and it replaces former FHA Documents A, B & C.

AIA DOCUMENT B352, DUTIES, RESPONSIBILITIES AND LIMITATIONS OF AUTHORITY OF THE ARCHITECT'S PROJECT REPRESENTATIVE

This document relates to the construction phase and is coordinated with AIA Document A201, *General Conditions of the Contract for Construction.* It should be attached to the owner-architect agreement as an exhibit when an architect's project representative is employed.

AIA DOCUMENT B431, ARCHITECT'S QUALIFICATION STATEMENT

The *Architect's Qualification Statement* may be used to set down in a clear, concise manner information relative to an architect's qualifications for performing architectural services for a specific project.

AIA DOCUMENT B727, STANDARD FORM OF AGREEMENT BETWEEN OWNER AND ARCHITECT FOR SPECIAL SERVICES

This is a standard form of agreement between owner and architect for special services, intended for use when other "B" series documents are not appropriate. It is often used for planning, feasibility studies, post-occupancy studies and other services that require a specialized description.

AIA DOCUMENT B801, STANDARD FORM OF AGREEMENT BETWEEN OWNER AND CONSTRUCTION MANAGER

This is a standard form of agreement between owner and construction manager. It is intended to be used with AIA Document B141/CM, *Standard Form of Agreement Between Owner and Architect, Construction Management Edition*, and AIA Document A201/CM, *General Conditions of the Contract for Construction, Construction Management Edition*.

The document is based on the premise that the owner will contract directly with multiple contractors for work, rather than through a general contractor or the construction manager.

The construction manager's services during the preconstruction phase are described, as are the owner's responsibilities and the responsibility for construction cost estimates.

C-SERIES

DOCUMENTS RELATING TO THE AGREEMENT BETWEEN THE ARCHITECT AND CONSULTANTS FOR PROFESSIONAL SERVICES.

AIA DOCUMENT C141, STANDARD FORM OF AGREEMENT BETWEEN ARCHITECT AND ENGINEER

This is a standard form of agreement between architect and engineer, establishing their responsibilities to each other and their mutual rights under the agreement. The document is most applicable to engineers providing services for architects who are providing the traditional five phases of "Basic Services" for owners under the provisions of AIA Document B141, *Owner-Architect Agreement*. Its provisions are in accord with those of B141 and of AIA Document A201, *General Conditions of the Contract for Construction*.

AIA DOCUMENT C161, STANDARD FORM OF AGREEMENT BETWEEN ARCHITECT AND ENGINEER FOR DESIGNATED SERVICES

This document is meant to be used in conjunction with the architect's use of AIA Document B161, *Owner-Architect Agreement for Designated Services*, and B162, *Scope of Designated Services*. The architect identifies the services that each consultant will perform under this agreement by marking them by a symbol in the column marked BY ARCHITECT AS OUTSIDE SERVICES in the owner-architect agreement, which must be attached to this agreement. This procedure allows the architect and engineer to conform their agreement to the owner-architect agreement for designated services.

AIA DOCUMENT C431, STANDARD FORM OF AGREEMENT BETWEEN ARCHITECT AND CONSULTANT FOR OTHER THAN NORMAL ENGINEERING SERVICES

This document is intended for use between the architect and a consultant for other than normal structural, mechanical or electrical engineering services. The consultant's services parallel the traditional five phases of services described in AIA Document B141, *Owner-Architect Agreement*.

AIA DOCUMENT C727, STANDARD FORM OF AGREEMENT BETWEEN ARCHITECT AND CONSULTANT FOR SPECIAL SERVICES

This is a standard form of agreement between architect and consultant for special services, intended for use when other "C" series documents are not appropriate. It is often used for planning, feasibility studies, post-occupancy studies and other services that require a specialized description.

AIA DOCUMENT C801, JOINT VENTURE AGREEMENT FOR PROFESSIONAL SERVICES

This document is intended to be used by two or more parties to provide for their mutual rights and obligations. It is intended that the joint venture, once established, will enter into a project agreement with the owner to provide professional services. The parties may be all architects, all engineers, a combination of architects and engineers, or other combination of professionals.

The document provides for selection between two methods of joint venture operations. The "Division of Compensation" method assumes that the services provided and the compensation received will be divided among the parties as agreed at the outset of the project. Each party's profitability is then dependent on individual performance and is not directly affected by performance of the other parties. The "Division of Profit/Loss" method is based on each party performing work and billing the joint venture at cost plus a nominal amount for overhead. The ultimate profit or loss of the joint venture is divided between the parties at the completion of the project.

D-SERIES

ARCHITECT-INDUSTRY DOCUMENTS.

AIA DOCUMENT D101, THE ARCHITECTURAL AREA AND VOLUME OF BUILDINGS

This document establishes definitions for and defines methods for calculating the architectural area and volume of buildings. The document also covers interstitial space, single occupant net assignable area and store net assignable area.

AIA DOCUMENT D200, PROJECT CHECKLIST

This is a convenient listing of tasks the practitioner normally would perform on a given project. The use of this checklist will assist the architect in recognizing the tasks required and in locating the data necessary to carry out assigned responsibilities. By providing space to note the date of actions taken, it may serve as a permanent record of the owner's, contractor's and architect's actions and decisions.

G-SERIES

CONTRACT AND OFFICE ADMINISTRATION FORMS.

AIA DOCUMENT G601, LAND SURVEY AGREEMENT

This is a standard form by which the owner requests a proposal and subsequently executes an agreement for surveying services. The form should be used in accordance with the owner-architect agreement provisions which establish the owner's responsibility for furnishing a certified survey of the site. The combination form enables the owner, in consultation with the architect, to establish the survey requirements for the site and to evaluate the proposal prior to executing the agreement.

AIA DOCUMENT G602, SOILS INVESTIGATION AND ENGINEERING SERVICES AGREEMENT (TEMPORARILY WITHDRAWN)

AIA DOCUMENT G604, CHANGE AUTHORIZATION FOR PROFESSIONAL SERVICES

This is a document intended to formalize procedures for authorizing supplemental professional actions such as expanding the scope of basic services, incurring reimbursable expenses or proceeding with certain additional services. The document should only be used in conjunction with an earlier agreement for professional services to provide a written record of such authorizations, giving particulars of activities, time spans and compensation involved. The document is flexible for use by any two parties, e.g., owner-architect, architect-engineer or other relationships.

AIA DOCUMENT G610, OWNER'S INSTRUCTIONS FOR BONDS AND INSURANCE

Since the owner, with the advice of insurance and legal counsel, should decide on the types and amounts of bonds and insurance the contractor will be required to carry and the insurance which the owner will carry, AIA Document G610 is a standard form which enables the architect to request written instructions from the owner concerning bonds and insurance.

AIA DOCUMENT G611, OWNER'S INSTRUCTIONS REGARDING BIDDING DOCUMENTS AND PROCEDURES

Since the owner, with advice of legal counsel, should decide on the requirements for the construction agreement and bidding procedures for the project, AIA Document G611 is a standard form which enables the architect to request written instructions from the owner regarding this information.

AIA DOCUMENT G701, CHANGE ORDER

A *Change Order* is the instrument by which changes in the work and adjustment in the contract sum or contract time under the owner-contractor agreement are formalized. The form provides a space for a complete description of the change, modifications to the contract sum, and adjustments in the contract time.

AIA DOCUMENT G701/CM, CHANGE ORDER– CONSTRUCTION MANAGEMENT EDITION

This document is essentially the same as the G701, *Change Order.* The major difference is that provision is made for the signature of the construction manager, who recommends to the architect and the owner that they, respectively, approve and authorize the Change Order.

AIA DOCUMENT G702, APPLICATION AND CERTIFICATE FOR PAYMENT; AIA DOCUMENT G703, CONTINUATION SHEET

These documents provide convenient and complete forms on which the contractor can make application for payment and on which the architect can certify that payment is due. The forms require the contractor to show the status of the contract sum to date including total dollar amount of work completed and stored to date, the amount of retainage, the total of previous payments, summary of change orders and the amount of current payment requested. G703, *Continuation Sheet,* breaks the contract sum into the portions of work in accordance with a schedule of values required by the general conditions. The form serves two purposes: contractor's application and architect's certification. Its use can expedite payment and reduce possibility of error. If the application is properly completed and acceptable to the architect, the architect's signature certifies to the owner that a payment in the amount indicated is due to the contractor. The form provides for the architect to certify

an amount different than the amount applied for, with explanation by the architect.

AIA DOCUMENT G704, CERTIFICATE OF SUBSTANTIAL COMPLETION

This is a standard form for recording the date of substantial completion of the work or designated portion thereof. The contractor prepares a list of items to be completed or corrected, and the architect verifies and amends this list. If the architect finds the work is substantially complete, a form is completed for acceptance by the contractor and the owner. Appended thereto is the list of items to be completed or corrected. The form provides for agreement as to the time allowed for completion or correction of the items, the date upon which the owner will occupy the work or designated portion thereof, and description of responsibilities for maintenance, heat, utilities, and insurance.

AIA DOCUMENT G705, CERTIFICATE OF INSURANCE

This is a standard form by which the contractor's insurors present to the owner a confirmation of insurance coverages relating to the project.

AIA DOCUMENT G706, CONTRACTOR'S AFFIDAVIT OF PAYMENT OF DEBTS AND CLAIMS

The contractor submits this affidavit with the final request for payment stating that all payrolls, bills for materials and equipment, and other indebtedness connected with the work for which the owner might be responsible have been paid or otherwise satisfied. The form requires that the contractor list specifically any indebtedness or known claims in connection with the construction contract which have not been paid or otherwise satisfied and to furnish a lien bond or indemnity bond to protect the owner with respect to each exception.

AIA DOCUMENT G706A, CONTRACTOR'S AFFIDAVIT OF RELEASE OF LIENS

This document supports AIA Document G706 in which the owner requires the contractor to submit releases or waivers of liens. In such cases, it is normal for the contractor to submit G706 duly executed, together with G706A duly executed with attached releases or waivers of liens for the contractor, all subcontractors and others who may have lien rights against the property of the owner. The contractor is required to list any exceptions to this statement and furnish a lien bond or indemnity bond to protect the owner with respect to such exceptions.

AIA DOCUMENT G707, CONSENT OF SURETY TO FINAL PAYMENT

By obtaining the surety's approval of final payment to the contractor and its agreement that final payment will not relieve the surety of any of its obligations, the owner may preserve its rights under the bonds.

AIA DOCUMENT G707A, CONSENT OF SURETY TO REDUCTION IN OR PARTIAL RELEASE OF RETAINAGE

This is a standard form for use when a surety company is involved with the project and the owner-contractor agreement contains a clause whereby retainage is reduced during the course of the construction project. The form, when duly executed, assures the owner that such reduction or partial release of retainage does not relieve the surety of its obligations.

AIA DOCUMENT G709, PROPOSAL REQUEST

This is a form used to secure price quotations which are necessary in the negotiation of change orders. The form is not a change order nor a direction to proceed with the work; it is simply a request to the contractor for information related to a proposed change in the construction contract.

AIA DOCUMENT G710, ARCHITECT'S SUPPLEMENTAL INSTRUCTIONS

Architect's Supplemental Instructions are used by the architect to issue supplemental instructions or interpretations or to order minor changes in the work. The form is intended to assist the architect in performing obligations as interpreter of the requirements of the contract documents in accordance with the owner-architect agreement and the general conditions of the contract. This form should not be used to change the contract sum or contract time. If the contractor believes that a change in contract sum or time is involved, different documents must be used.

AIA DOCUMENT G711, ARCHITECT'S FIELD REPORT

The *Architect's Field Report* is a standard form for the architect's project representative to use to maintain a concise record of site visits or, in case of a full time project representative, a daily log of construction activities.

AIA DOCUMENT G712, SHOP DRAWING AND SAMPLE RECORD

This is a standard form by which the architect can schedule and monitor shop drawings and samples. Since this process tends to be a complicated one, this schedule, showing the progress of a submittal, is an aid in the orderly processing of work and will serve as a permanent record of the chronology of this process.

AIA DOCUMENT G713, CONSTRUCTION CHANGE AUTHORIZATION

This is an authorization form for immediate changes in the work which, if not processed expeditiously, might delay the project. These changes are often initiated in the field and usually affect the contract sum or the contract time. This is not a change order, but only an authorization to proceed with a change for subsequent inclusion in a change order. It establishes a basis for change in time or cost.

AIA DOCUMENT G722, PROJECT APPLICATION AND PROJECT CERTIFICATE FOR PAYMENT; AIA DOCUMENT G723, PROJECT APPLICATION SUMMARY

These documents have a purpose similar to that of the combination of G702, *Application and Certificate for Payment,* and G703, *Continuation Sheet,* but are for use on construction management projects.

Each contractor submits a separate G702, *Application and Certificate for Payment,* to the construction manager who compiles them to complete the G723, *Project Application Summary.* Project totals are then transferred to a G722, *Project Application and Project Certificate for Payment.* The construction manager can then sign the form, have it notarized and submit it with the G723 (which has all of the separate contractors' G702 forms attached) to the architect for review and appropriate action.

Appendix C

GLOSSARY OF LABORATORY TERMINOLOGY

APPENDIX C • GLOSSARY OF LABORATORY TERMINOLOGY

A

Acid-fast organisms—Bacteria that retain aniline stains so tenaciously that it is not decolorized by 5 percent mineral acids. Examples of acid-fast organisms are *Mycobacterium tuberculosis* causing tuberculosis and *Mycobacterium leprae* causing leprosy.

Anemia—A condition in which the red corpuscles of the blood are reduced in number or deficient in hemoglobin.

Antibiotic sensitivity—Method used by the laboratory to determine susceptibility of a microorganism to an antimicrobial agent.

Antibodies—A protein substance (immunoglobulin) in tissue or body fluids which acts in antagonism to specific foreign bodies (antigens).

Antigen—A substance, usually a protein, which when introduced into the body stimulates the production of an antibody.

Autoclaves—An apparatus for sterilizing by superheated steam under pressure.

B

Bacteria—A large, widely distributed group of typically one-celled microorganisms, many of which are disease-producing. These are detected in the area labeled "bacti" or bacteriology.

Blood bank—Function of this section is to collect, process, preserve, prepare, and distribute blood and blood components to provide safe transfusions of blood products to patients.

Blood cells—Formed elements of the blood divided into red blood cells (erythrocytes) and white blood cells (leukocytes).

Blood fractions—Whole blood is blood from which none of the elements have been removed. Blood can be separated into many components (fractions) such as the liquid portion (plasma), red blood cells, white blood cells, platelets, and various coagulation factors.

Blood gas—The measurement of the partial pressures (pCO_2, pO_2) exerted by the dissolved oxygen and carbon dioxide in the blood. Blood pH has become a universally accepted companion of pCO_2 and pO_2 measurement.

C

Calculi—Abnormal concretions occurring within the body, usually composed of mineral salts.

Cell washers—An instrument commonly used in the blood bank that uses a centrifuge to wash, decant, mix, and rewash cells automatically.

Celloidin specimens—A tissue specimen embedded in celloidin, which is a purified form of nitrocellulose. Celloidin is used as a supporting medium for tissues so that the tissues can be sectioned.

Cerebrospinal fluid—The fluid contained within the ventricles of the brain and surrounding the brain and spinal cord in the subarachnoid space.

Clinical chemistry—That scientific discipline which performs qualitative and quantitative chemical analyses of body fluids such as blood, urine, spinal fluid, feces, and other materials.

Coagulation—The sequential process by which the multiple coagulation factors of the blood interact, ultimately resulting in the formation of an insoluble blood clot.

Coagulation concentrates—Plasma derivatives containing high levels of coagulation factors used to treat coagulation factor deficiencies, i.e., AHG concentrate.

Colony counting—A calibrated amount of urine is inoculated upon culture media and after a proper incubation, the number of colonies that grow is estimated and reported as a measure of the degree of bacteria present in the sample.

229

Component therapy—Transfusion of only the indicated portion of blood which is separated from the whole blood by physical or mechanical means.

CO_2—Carbon dioxide, an odorless, colorless gas resulting from oxidation of carbon. It is formed in the tissues and eliminated by the lungs.

Cross-matching—Tests performed on both the blood to be transfused and the blood of the prospective recipient to insure absence of incompatibility.

Cryoprecipitate—The cold insoluble precipitate remaining when fresh frozen plasma is thawed at 4°C. There is a high concentration of antihemophilic factor.

Culturing—The propagation of microorganisms in or on special media conducive to their growth.

Cytocentrifuging—The process where cells are separated from their suspension medium and recovered on a microslide as the specimen's suspension medium is absorbed by a blotter. Cytocentrifugation is performed in a bench-top centrifuge with a specially designed rotor and sample chambers.

Cytologic studies—Microscopic examination of cells desquamated from a body surface commonly used as a means of detecting malignant change.

Cytology—The study of cell structure as a screening method for possible malignancy.

D

Decalcification—The process of removing calcareous matter from bone.

DIC—See disseminated intravascular coagulation

Differential—Pertaining to the differential blood count, a method of counting the percentage of different types of white blood cells in a smear.

Disseminated intravascular coagulation—Abnormal clotting of blood within the vessels of the body.

E

Electron microscope—An instrument used to obtain an enlarged image of small objects and reveal details of structure not otherwise distinguishable using an electron beam to form an image for viewing on a fluorescent screen.

Embedding—The fixation of tissue specimen in a firm medium, in order to keep it intact during the cutting of thin sections.

Etiologic—Pertaining to etiology, the study or theory of the factors that cause disease and the method of their introduction to the host.

F

Feces—The excrement discharged from the intestines, consisting of bacteria, cells exfoliated from the intestines, secretions and a small amount of food residue.

Fixative solutions—Agents used in the preparation of a histologic or pathologic specimen for the purpose of maintaining the existing form and structure of all its constituent elements.

Flame photometer—An instrument for analyzing the light emitted by a substance in a flame.

Fluorescent microscopy—Examination under or observation by means of a microscope of natural fluorescent materials or of specimens stained with fluorochromes, which emit light when exposed to blue or ultraviolet light.

Formaldehyde—A powerful disinfectant gas formerly used as a disinfectant. A 37 percent solution of formaldehyde gas in water (formalin) is widely used in fixing fluid for pathologic specimens or as a preservative. Dilutions have also been used as a surgical and general antiseptic and as an astringent.

Frozen sections—A section cut by a microtome for tissue that has been frozen and used for rapid diagnosis during surgery.

Fungi—Plural of fungus, a general term used to denote a group of eukaryotic protists, including mushrooms, yeasts, rusts, molds, smuts, etc., which are characterized by the absence of chlorophyll and by the presence of a rigid cell wall composed of chitin, mannans, and sometimes cellulose. They are usually of simple morphological form or show some reversible cellular specialization.

G

Gas chromatography—A method of chemical analysis in which an inert gas is used to move the vapors of the materials to be separated through a column of inert material (or stationary phase). The different solutes move through the stationary phase at different velocities according to their degree of attraction to it, producing separated compounds.

Gram-negative sepsis—The presence in the blood or other tissues of gram-negative microorganisms or their toxins. Gram-negative organisms lose stain or are decolorized by alcohol in Gram's method of staining.

H

Hematology—That branch of medical science which studies the morphology of blood and blood-forming tissues.

Histopathology—The area of anatomy which deals with the minute structure, composition, and function of diseased tissues.

Hot air sterilization—The complete elimination of microbial viability by means of hot air.

I

Immunodiffusion—The diffusion of antigen and antibody from separate reservoirs to form decreasing concentration gradients in hydrophilic gels.

Immunoelectrophoresis—A method of combining electrophoresis and double diffusion for distinguishing between proteins and other materials by means of their electrophoretic mobility and antigenic specificities. In general, the antigen is placed in a central well and subjected to electrophoresis. The antibody is then placed in rectangular wells which are parallel to the direction of the electrophoresis. Double diffusion occurs between the antibody in the rectangular wells and the antigen.

Immunology—That branch of biomedical science concerned with the response of the organism to antigenic challenge, the recognition of self from not self, and all the biological (in vivo), serological (in vitro), and physical chemical aspects of immune phenomena.

In vitro—Reactions or processes occurring in an artificial environment, i.e., in a test tube.

In vivo—Reactions or processes occurring within the body.

Incubation—Holding media growth plates at constant temperature to favor growth of microorganisms or tissue culture.

Intracellular organism—Any living thing inside a cell or cells.

L

Leukocytosis—An abnormally large number of white blood cells in the blood.

M

Media—A substance used for the cultivation (growth) of microorganisms such as bacteria.

Micro procedures—(1) Usually refers to microbiology procedures. (2) Culture (growth) and antibiotic sensitivity tests done in a microbiology laboratory.

Microbiology—A clinical laboratory section or division which identifies microorganisms.

Microorganism—Any microscopic living thing.

Microscopic—Visible only through a microscope.

Microtome—A slicing instrument for cutting thin sections from tissue to study under a microscope.

Millipore filter techniques—Filtering material used usually with a vacuum to remove microorganisms from liquids.

N

Nuclear medicine—(1) The clinical use of radioactive material to produce images for diagnostic evaluation. (2) A laboratory division using radioactive material in testing to determine substances in medically important specimens.

P

Packed cell volume—Also called hematocrit or micro-hematocrit. The percent of total-blood volume occupied by the cells after centrifugation.

Papanicolaou technique—The cytological examination of material taken from a female cervix to detect possible cancer.

Paraffin blocks—Tissue specimens imbedded in paraffin cubes in preparation for microtome slicing.

Parasites—Organisms that live in or on another organism and get their nourishment from the host.

Parasitology preparation—The material prepared by centrifugation which is placed on a slide for microscopic examination.

pH—A logarithmic scale used to express the acidity of blood and urine specimens.

Phlebotomy—The collection of blood specimens by venipuncture, skin puncture, or arterial puncture.

Plasma—The fluid or noncellular portion of blood.

Plasma expellers—Mechanical jaw-like device for squeezing a blood bag to push plasma out the top and thus separate it from the packed cells.

Plasmapheresis—A procedure in which blood is removed from the body in order to separate cells and plasma and then return the cells without the plasma proteins to the body.

Platelet—A small irregularly shaped cell in blood which is involved in the clotting process.

R

Radioactivity—The property of some atoms to spontaneously emit rays or subatomic particles with the release of energy.

Radionuclide—Any atom which has radioactive properties.

Raw count—The actual counts recorded by an instrument measuring emissions from radioactive substances. These numbers are corrected for simultaneous emissions and other factors to calculate the true count.

Rectilinear scanner—A device used to convert gamma rays into electrical impulses which when magnified are registered on x-ray film or as dots on scan paper. A motor-driven detector moves automatically in a linear fashion across the area being examined.

Red blood cell—One of the cellular elements of peripheral blood, an erythrocyte. The mature form is a nonnucleated biconcave disc.

Routine—A term used to describe a common or usual situation in regard to a procedure or circumstance.

S

Scintillation gamma camera—A device used to detect the presence of gamma ray emissions. Slight variations in radiation intensity may be identified without the need to follow a direct-linear function.

Serologic studies—Analytical studies pertaining to serology.

Serology—The study of in-vitro antigen-antibody reactions.

Single probe with collimator—A device-forming part of a nuclear scanning instrument which defines the area from which gamma rays emanate. Usually formed of lead, the collimator extends out from the crystal of the detection unit.

Special—A term used to describe an unusual event or circumstance, or a procedure used to detect biologic properties which are uncommon or not normally identified.

Spinal fluid—That clear biologic fluid which surrounds the spinal cord.

Staining—The process of exposing biologic material to special dyes for the purpose of identification of cellular detail.

STAT—An abbreviation of a Latin word meaning immediately, usually referring to a request for an analysis in an emergent situation.

Sterilization—A process concerned with the elimination of microbial viability.

Streak—A linear growth of a specific microorganism used to enhance the viability of adjacent elements of diagnostic significance.

Subculturing—The technique used in selection of specific colonies of microorganisms from a culture surface supporting a wide variety of growth.

T

Toxicology—The study of poisons including detection and quantitative analysis as well as the management of related clinical disorders.

Turbidity—A term used to describe the presence of a cloudy appearance in fluid material.

Typing—A method of measuring tissue or blood compatibility between two individuals or of showing differences in the characteristics of some microorganisms.

U

Ultrastructure—The arrangement of the smallest elements of the cell and supporting tissue; structure beyond the range of the light microscope.

Urinalysis—The physical, chemical, and microscopic analysis of urine.

V

Virology—That branch of microbiology concerned with the study of viruses and viral diseases.

Viruses—A group of minute microorganisms undetectable by light microscopy and characterized by the lack of an independent metabolism.

W

Water baths—Items of laboratory equipment designed to maintain water at a constant temperature.

Water demineralization—The process of removal of excessive or unwanted mineral or organic salts from water used in laboratory analysis.

White blood cell—One of the cellular elements of peripheral blood, a leucocyte. Divided into six types the mature forms vary as to size, nuclear structure, and cytoplasmic granulation.

Appendix D

CONSTRUCTION SPECIFICATIONS
INSTITUTE INDEX

CONSTRUCTION SPECIFICATIONS INSTITUTE INDEX

Division 1–GENERAL REQUIREMENTS

01001	General conditions
01010	General requirements
01311	Network analysis system
01340	Samples and shop drawings
01410	Testing laboratory services
01568	Environmental protection
01569	Asbestos removal

Division 2–SITEWORK

02050	Demolition
02200	Earthwork
02201	Earthwork (short form)
02210	Grading
02240	Soil stabilization (erosion control)
02360	Foundation piles
02362	Auger placed concrete piles
02370	Foundation caissons
02411	Foundation drainage
02441	Lawn irrigation system
02444	Chain link fences and gate
02446	Special fences (ornamental metal, decorative wood and environmental)
02452	Exterior signage
02470	Site furnishings (benches, game tables, planters, tree gates, trash receptacles, and other site crafts)
02480	Landscaping
02513	Asphaltic concrete paving
02514	Unit pavers
02515	Site work concrete
02577	Pavement marking
02710	Distribution and transmission system (steam)
02711	Gas system
02713	Water system
02720	Storm and sanitary sewerage system

Division 3–CONCRETE

03300	Cast-in-place concrete
03301	Cast-in-place concrete (short form)
03412	Precast concrete roofing slab
03450	Architectural precast concrete panels
03512	Roof decks, cast-in-place gypsum
03532	Cement-fiber roof deck

Division 4–MASONRY

04200	Unit masonry
04230	Reinforced unit masonry
04435	Cast stone

Division 5–METALS

05120	Structural steel
05210	Steel joists
05311	Steel decking
05321	Steel decking composite
05500	Metal fabrication
05510	Metal stairs
05805	Expansion joint covers

Division 6–WOOD AND PLASTIC

06100	Rough carpentry
06200	Finish carpentry and millwork

Division 7–THERMAL AND MOISTURE PROTECTION

07112	Bituminous membrane waterproofing (built-up)
07113	Modified bituminous membrane waterproofing (sheet)

07114	Shower pan waterproofing
07140	Metal oxide waterproofing
07160	Bituminous dampproofing
07210	Building insulation
07211	Loose fill insulation
07220	Insulation concrete
07221	Insulating concrete composite (for concrete deck)
07222	Insulation concrete composite (for metal deck)
07250	Firestopping
07253	Sprayed-on fireproofing (mineral fiber)
07311	Asphalt shingles
07314	Slate shingles
07321	Clay roofing tiles
07410	Preformed wall and roof panels
07440	Preformed plastic panels
07510	Built-up roofing and roof insulation
07540	Fluid applied roofing (over sprayed urethane)
07541	Fluid applied roofing (over concrete)
07550	inverted roofing system
07570	Elastomeric coating (pedestrian traffic)
07571	Latex mastic deck covering
07600	Flashing and sheet metal
07610	Batten seam roofing
07800	Roof accessories
07920	Sealants and caulking

Division 8–DOORS AND WINDOWS

08110	Steel doors and frames
08210	Wood doors
08305	Access doors
08310	Sliding metal fire doors
08331	Overhead coiling doors
08341	Overhead rolling shutters
08353	Accordion folding doors
08355	Flexible door
08410	Aluminum entrances and store fronts
08450	Revolving doors
08510	Steel windows (double hung)
08520	Aluminum windows (single/double/triple/hung)

08522	Pivoted aluminum windows (double glazed)
08523	Projected aluminum windows
08524	Side hinged aluminum windows (double glazed)
08525	Horizontal sliding aluminum windows
08526	Casement aluminum windows
08527	Aluminum jalousie windows
08529	Aluminum storm windows (triple track self storing)
08710	Builders' hardware
08730	Weatherstripping and seals
08810	Glass and glazing

Division 9–FINISHES

09050	Color design
09200	Lathing and gypsum plastering
09205	Lathing and cement plastering
09215	Veneer plaster
09260	Gypsum wallboard systems
09310	Ceramic tile
09410	Portland cement terrazzo
09421	Terrazzo tile
09500	Acoustical treatment
09600	Stone and brick flooring
09660	Resilient tile flooring
09660	Resilient sheet flooring
09666	Resilient sheet flooring (heat welded seam)
09682	Carpeting (without cushion)
09690	Carpet module
09695	Soft surface flooring
09701	Latex mastic flooring
09731	Conductive elastomeric flooring
09815	High-build glazed coatings
09900	Painting
09951	Vinyl coated fabric wall covering

Division 10–SPECIALTIES

10100	Chalkboards and tackboards
10152	Hospital cubical curtains and intravenous support tracks

10162	Metal toilet partitions and urinal screens
10170	Prefabricated shower/and dressing/ compartments
10200	Louvers and wall vents
10260	Wall bumpers and corner guards
10270	Access flooring
10350	Flagpoles
10360	Miscellaneous specialties
10440	Signs (interior)
10500	Lockers
10522	Fire extinguisher cabinets
10551	Mail chutes
10552	Mail boxes
10601	Mesh partitions
10617	Moveable metal partitions
10623	Accordion folding partitions
10650	Scales
10671	Metal storage shelving
10800	Toilet and bath accessories

Division 11—EQUIPMENT

11021	Vault doors and day gates
11022	Service window units—bullet resistant
11052	Library shelving, steel
11131	Projection screen
11150	Parking controls
11160	Loading dock equipment
11171	Package incinerator
11192	Detention and projection screens
11401	Custom fabricated food service equipment
11410	Food service cooking equipment
11411	Food service warewashing equipment
11412	Food waste machines
11415	Food service self-contained refrigeration equipment
11416	Food service equipment—utility distribution system
11420	Food service grease extracting ventilators
11450	Residential equipment
11451	Kitchen equipment

11460	Unit kitchen—type 22
11461	Nourishment unit—type 22E
11471	Revolving darkroom doors
11475	Photographic processing equipment
11491	Hydrotherapy equipment
11602	Laboratory accessories
11604	Biohazard safety cabinets
11610	Laboratory fume hoods
11612	Water distribution equipment
11614	Laboratory washing equipment
11615	Laboratory controlled temperature rooms
11620	Custom fabricated laboratory equipment
11701	Solution warming cabinets
11710	Sterilizer and associated equipment
11712	Hospital washing equipment
11781	Autopsy tables

Division 12—FURNISHINGS

12301	Metal casework
12302	Wood casework
12336	Medication cabinet
12340	Pharmacy furniture
12345	Laboratory furniture
12351	Nurse server
12501	Drapery hardware
12513	Window shades
12514	Lightproof shades
12645	Ecclesiastical furniture

Division 13—SPECIAL CONSTRUCTION

13062	Walk-in refrigerators and freezers
13091	Lead radiation shielding
13121	Pre-engineered metal buildings
13154	Therapeutic pool accessories
13171	Chain link animal enclosures
13412	Elevated water tank
13980	Solar energy collection systems

Division 14–CONVEYING SYSTEMS

14105	Dumbwaiters (automatic loading and unloading)
14450	Motor vehicle lifts
14560	Chutes (linen and trash)
14581	Pneumatic tube system
14582	Pneumatic soil linen and trash system

Division 15–MECHANICAL

15050	Basic methods and requirements (mechanical)
15051	Basic requirements and methods (boiler plant)
15139	Pump (plumbing)
15140	Pumps (HVAC)
15200	Noise and vibration control
15201	Noise and vibration control and seismic requirements (boiler plant)
15250	Insulation
15262	Boiler plant insulation
15311	Compressed air systems
15312	Oxygen system
15313	Vacuum system
15315	Nitrous oxide system
15317	Nitrogen system
15318	Oral evacuation system
15319	Compressed air system, shop and laundry
15321	Dental compressed air system
15339	Boiler plant piping systems
15346	Oil and gasoline installation
15371	Water softening system
15372	Water dealkalizing system
15400	Plumbing systems
15424	Domestic water heaters
15450	Plumbing fixtures and trim
15460	Therapeutic pool equipment
15501	Wet automatic sprinkler system
15530	Standpipe and hose system
15606	Oil storage tanks (boiler plant)
15614	Boiler breechings and stacks
15622	Fire tube boilers and accessories
15624	Water tube steam boilers and accessories
15625	Boiler plant mechanical equipment
15650	Refrigeration equipment (HVAC)
15651	Refrigerant piping
15680	Cooling tower
15704	Water treatment (HVAC)
15705	HVAC piping systems
15706	Preinsulated chilled water piping
15740	Terminal units
15750	Heating and cooling coils
15763	Air handling units
15770	Unitary air-conditioning equipment
15819	Energy recovery equipment
15822	Fans
15840	Ductwork and accessories
15880	Air filters
15900	Controls and instrumentation
15901	Controls and instrumentation (boiler plant)
15920	Extension of existing engineering control center (ECC)
15921	Engineering control center (ECC)—class A
15922	Engineering control center (ECC)—class B
15923	Engineering control center (ECC)—class C
15924	Engineering control center (ECC)—class D
15980	Testing, adjusting, and balancing

Division 16–ELECTRICAL

16050	Basic methods and requirements (electrical)
16051	Electrical systems protective device study
16111	Conduit systems
16112	Busway
16113	Underfloor ducts
16126	Cables, high voltage (above 600 V)
16127	Cables low voltage (600 V and below)
16140	Wiring devices
16150	Motors

16155	Motor starters
16160	Panelboards
16170	Disconnects (motor and circuit)
16208	Engine generators
16251	Automatic transfer switches
16312	Unit substation, secondary
16320	Transformers
16321	Transformers padmounted
16361	Switchgear, high voltage (above 600 V)
16362	Switches, high voltage (above 600 V)
16402	Underground electrical construction
16430	Metering
16450	Grounding
16460	Transformers (general purpose)
16461	Transformers (specialty)
16462	Distribution switchboard
16464	Switchgear, low voltage (600 V and below)
16510	Building lighting, interior
16530	Site lighting
16601	Lighting protection system
16640	Cathodic protection (boiler plant systems)
16665	Miscellaneous medical construction
16670	Radiology electrical systems
16675	Isolated power systems
16680	Medical and surgical lighting fixtures
16685	Patient wall systems
16690	Intensive care monitor modules
16721	Fire alarm—local building system
16722	Fire alarm—base loop system
16726	Medical gas alarms
16727	Ultrasonic motion detector (UMD)
16760	Intercommunication systems
16761	Audio-visual call and code one system
16762	Dental clinic intercommunication and patient annunciation system
16770	Public address system
16771	Radio entertainment distribution system
16772	Radio entertainment extension system
16781	Master TV antenna equipment
16782	Master TV antenna equipment and systems extension
16920	Motor control centers
16921	Motor control panelboards

Appendix E

DEMOGRAPHICS, SPACE, WORKLOAD, AND PERSONNEL

DEMOGRAPHICS, SPACE, WORKLOAD, AND PERSONNEL

A Survey of 201 American Laboratories

This appendix contains data gathered in 1984 from 201 American laboratories. In this appendix data are correlated by six basic laboratory types and sizes, and the correlated data are broken down by laboratory sections. Regression curves relating section test performing space in square feet to CAP Workload Units and personnel FTEs are shown at the end of this appendix. The Laboratory Function and Design Committee is not aware of any similar published data of such a comprehensive nature.

The reader is cautioned that the data are only a compilation of representative laboratories in the United States and are most specifically not a method of deriving space requirements. The data may be useful for comparative purposes. Each laboratory should be designed to meet the particular needs of its service area.

A. S. KOENIG, M.D., *Editor*

In 1984 THE CAP LABORATORY FUNCTION AND DESIGN COMMITTEE undertook a survey of American laboratories. The purposes of this survey include the following: The committee wished to see how much similarity existed between laboratories of different types. Also, the committee wished to test the validity of several methods that have been used throughout the years for deriving space requirements. Lastly, the committee desired to provide pathologists and architects with a data base of material that could be used for comparative purposes in the planning and design process.

Because of the diversity of laboratories and the manner in which each keeps its statistics, an effort was made to gather as "clean" a data base as possible. Since the CAP Computer Assisted Workload Recording Program and CAP Surveys program impose a uniform statistical recording method, laboratories were selected that participated in one or both programs. All laboratories agreed to participate on a voluntary basis for this survey.

Despite this selection, not all laboratories were able to provide all of the

243

information requested. In some areas where responses were not given, the committee was required to make assumptions, e.g., changing responses from zero to missing in some instances, and from missing to zero in others. Where these occur, it is the committee's belief that the data were enhanced. Two computer runs were made on the data by the CAP Computer Center resulting in a 293-page printout of tables, regressions, correlations, scatter plots, and histograms. The material that follows represents the highlights of this information.

Demographic Information

The 201 laboratories were divided into six basic groups depending on ownership and/or bed size. The distribution of these groups is depicted in Figure E.1. The bed size of each of these groups expressed in median and percentiles follows in Figure E.2. These data include bassinets.

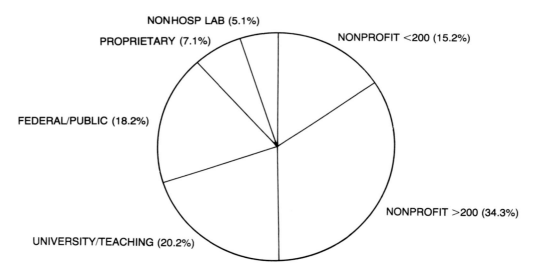

Fig. E.1 LABORATORY TYPES BY OWNERSHIP
Distribution by Laboratory Type

NONHOSP LAB (5.1%)
PROPRIETARY (7.1%)
NONPROFIT <200 (15.2%)
FEDERAL/PUBLIC (18.2%)
NONPROFIT >200 (34.3%)
UNIVERSITY/TEACHING (20.2%)

The total patient days for each institution are as follows in Figure E.3. When comparing your laboratory with others, it is of interest how new the laboratories in the comparative group are. This is depicted for all laboratories and broken down by type in Figures E.4 and E.5. For example, if a laboratory was built or remodeled between 1975 and 1980 it will show in the 1980 column.

244

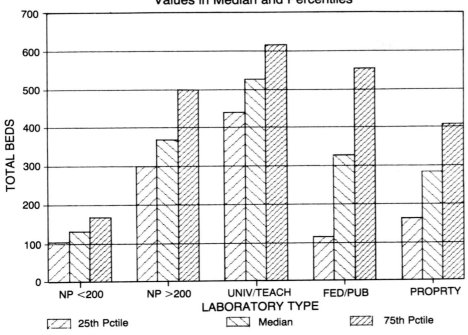

Fig. E.2   BED SIZE OF PARTICIPATING LABORATORIES
Values in Median and Percentiles

The total patient days are as follows:

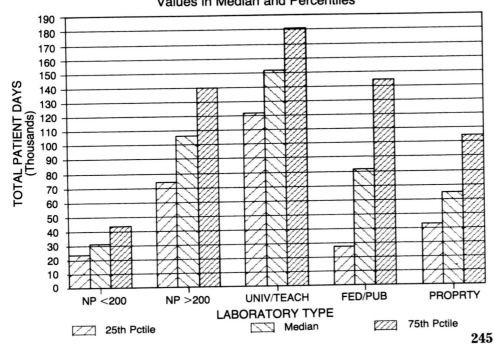

Fig. E.3   TOTAL PATIENT DAYS
Values in Median and Percentiles

245

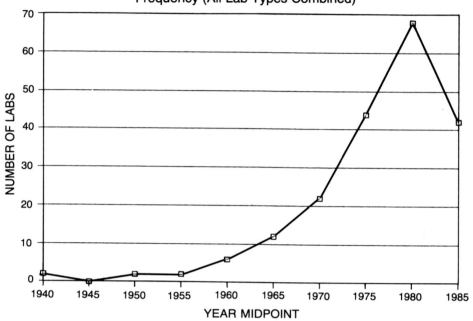

Fig. E.4 YEAR LAB BUILT OR REMODELED
Frequency (All Lab Types Combined)

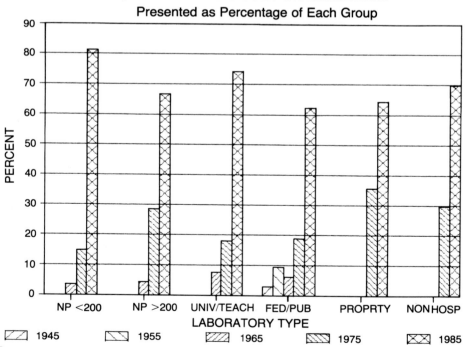

Fig. E.5 YEAR LAB BUILT OR REMODELED
Presented as Percentage of Each Group

246

In some cases laboratories may be located on multiple floors. This may depend on service requirements or more commonly on physical constraints of the building. The occurrence of this on a percentage basis is depicted in Figure E.6.

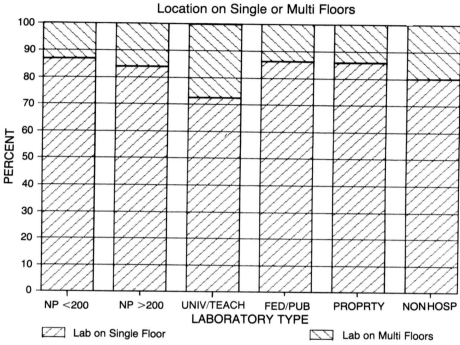

Fig. E.6 LOCATION OF MAIN LABORATORY
Location on Single or Multi Floors

Many laboratories may have satellite or special function laboratories that are separate from the main laboratory area. The existence of these facilities is costly in duplication of equipment and personnel. However, because of special service requirements or distance from the main laboratory area, they may be requested. The occurrence of these on a percentage basis is shown in Figure E.7.

Usually satellite or special function laboratories are quite small and are linked administratively to the main laboratory facility. The mean square footage of some of the more common of these laboratories is shown in Figure E.8. In this example all laboratory groups are combined. The mean of personnel for these laboratories is shown in Figure E.9.

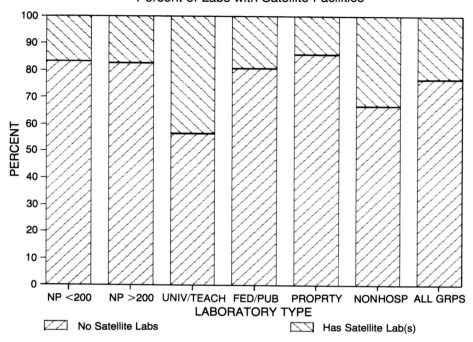

Fig. E.7   SATELLITE AND SPECIAL FUNCTION LABS
Percent of Labs with Satellite Facilities

PERCENT

LABORATORY TYPE

[ ] No Satellite Labs   [ ] Has Satellite Lab(s)

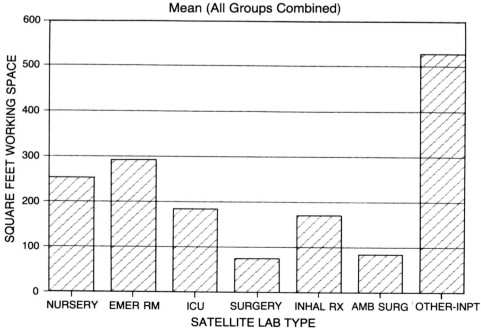

Fig. E.8   SQ FT IN SATELLITE LABS
Mean (All Groups Combined)

SQUARE FEET WORKING SPACE

SATELLITE LAB TYPE

248

Fig. E.9 FTE PERSONNEL IN SATELLITE LABS
Mean (All Groups Combined)

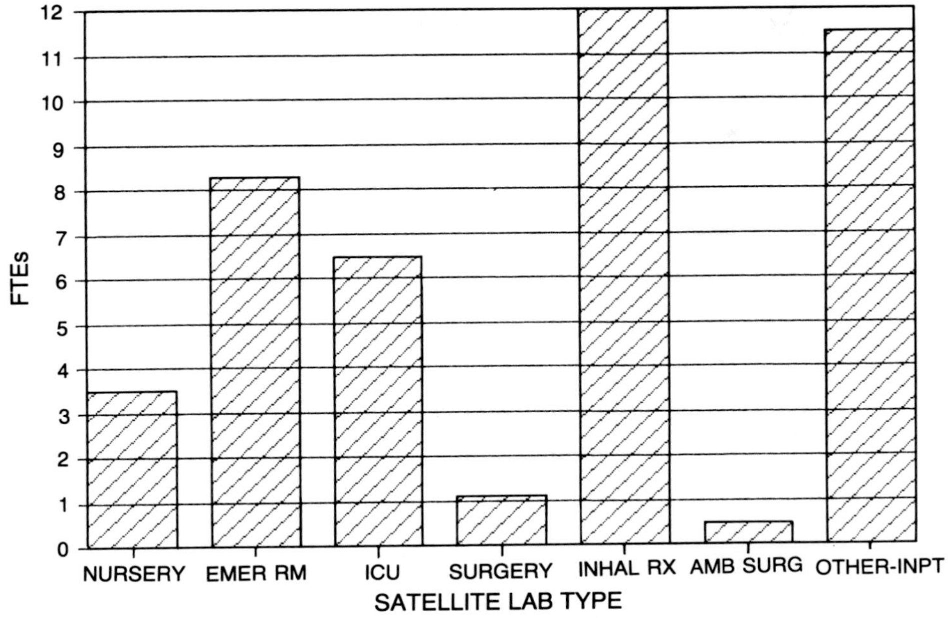

Laboratory Area (space)

In addition to actual square feet, each survey participant was asked to estimate the required square feet they believed necessary to comfortably handle their current workload. It is common to hear the complaint that not enough work space is available in the laboratory. In all groups the required square footage was larger than actual square footage. However, the median difference was surprisingly small in most cases. The values given in Figure E.10 represent only the SUM of individual section work space. They do not include hallways, administrative areas, offices, etc. Each laboratory was also asked to estimate the total square feet that would be required in five years. This value is also shown in Figure E.10.

Comparisons of actual and required space on a section by section basis among different laboratory types are shown in Table E.1. The values are expressed in medians and percentiles. Table E.2 shows the same breakdowns expressed in percentages of total work area space for Clinical Pathology space and Anatomic Pathology space. In this case the percentages do not total 100 percent because the different number of respondents in each laboratory type were calculated separately. However, in most cases they are reasonably close.

249

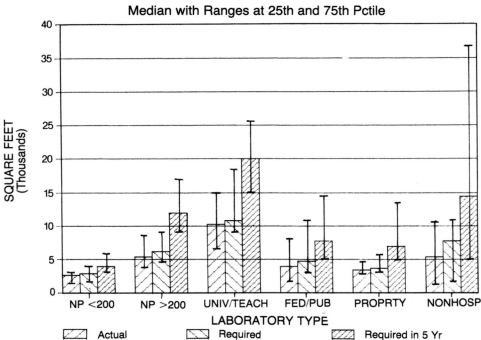

Fig. E.10 TOTAL TEST—AREA SPACE IN SQUARE FEET
Median with Ranges at 25th and 75th Pctile

Nontest areas of the laboratory may vary tremendously in size and availability. Each of these areas should be designed to meet the needs of each laboratory. Administrative and other nontest areas are similar in size to those found in standard office settings and should meet the same needs. Table E.3 shows the distribution and need for most of the nontest areas that may occur in the laboratory setting. All laboratory types are combined in this table.

A number of factors are recognized that impact on laboratory space needs. The survey participants were asked to express an opinion on how some of the more significant factors might change their space needs in the forseeable future. Their responses, grouped by laboratory type, are given in Table E.4.

Table E.1

LABORATORY TEST PERFORMANCE AREAS IN SQ FT
ACTUAL AND REQUIRED SQ FOOTAGES

	Actual 25th	Actual Median	Actual 75th	Required 25th	Required Median	Required 75th

● CLINICAL PATHOLOGY WORK AREAS

——————————————— LAB AREA—BLOOD BANK ———————————————

	Actual 25th	Actual Median	Actual 75th	Required 25th	Required Median	Required 75th
NONPROFIT <200	101.0	156.0	260.0	150.0	232.0	297.3
NONPROFIT >200	282.8	425.5	647.5	336.3	537.0	806.8
UNIV/TEACH	500.0	652.0	1,231.0	700.0	900.0	1,300.0
FEDERAL/PUBLIC	146.0	288.0	575.0	151.0	320.0	787.5
PROPRIETARY	187.0	220.0	435.0	187.0	350.0	450.0
NONHOSPITAL	70.0	1,104.0	1,277.0	70.0	1,530.0	1,733.0

——————————————— LAB AREA—CHEMISTRY ———————————————

	Actual 25th	Actual Median	Actual 75th	Required 25th	Required Median	Required 75th
NONPROFIT <200	450.0	612.0	930.0	500.0	624.0	1,100.0
NONPROFIT >200	940.5	1,330.0	2,067.0	1,102.8	1,500.0	2,281.3
UNIV/TEACH	1,413.8	2,245.0	3,158.5	1,661.0	2,650.0	3,428.0
FEDERAL/PUBLIC	567.0	943.0	1,820.0	800.0	1,400.0	2,700.0
PROPRIETARY	575.0	1,064.0	1,351.0	750.0	1,064.0	1,600.0
NONHOSPITAL	436.5	1,713.0	3,345.5	736.5	2,000.0	4,119.5

——————————————— LAB AREA—HEMATOLOGY/COAGULATION ———————————————

	Actual 25th	Actual Median	Actual 75th	Required 25th	Required Median	Required 75th
NONPROFIT <200	152.0	225.0	285.8	201.0	262.5	404.5
NONPROFIT >200	415.5	556.5	786.8	457.5	700.0	1,000.0
UNIV/TEACH	735.0	1,028.0	1,375.5	800.8	1,188.0	1,630.5
FEDERAL/PUBLIC	260.0	437.0	672.0	300.0	564.0	1,000.0
PROPRIETARY	138.0	330.0	644.0	195.0	540.0	713.0
NONHOSPITAL	137.3	312.5	620.8	195.8	312.5	590.0

——————————————— LAB AREA—IMMUNOLOGY ———————————————

	Actual 25th	Actual Median	Actual 75th	Required 25th	Required Median	Required 75th
NONPROFIT <200	27.5	78.5	180.8	47.5	126.5	200.0
NONPROFIT >200	100.0	192.0	329.5	147.0	240.0	430.0
UNIV/TEACH	204.0	416.0	760.0	243.5	631.0	1,000.0
FEDERAL/PUBLIC	100.0	164.5	381.8	100.0	200.0	262.5
PROPRIETARY	108.0	136.0	252.0	135.0	252.0	500.0
NONHOSPITAL	128.3	338.0	625.0	218.8	368.5	660.5

——————————————— LAB AREA—MICROBIOLOGY ———————————————

	Actual 25th	Actual Median	Actual 75th	Required 25th	Required Median	Required 75th
NONPROFIT <200	150.0	248.0	406.3	200.0	300.0	514.0
NONPROFIT >200	500.0	745.0	1,115.0	647.5	912.0	1,375.0
UNIV/TEACH	834.0	1,274.0	2,050.0	1,000.0	1,400.0	2,600.0
FEDERAL/PUBLIC	344.0	576.0	1,440.0	434.0	833.0	1,602.0
PROPRIETARY	372.5	500.0	844.5	372.5	650.0	998.0
NONHOSPITAL	150.0	805.0	2,803.8	414.5	876.0	2,938.8

(continued)

Table E.1 (continued)	Actual 25th	Actual Median	Actual 75th	Required 25th	Required Median	Required 75th
LAB AREA—RADIOISOTOPES						
NONPROFIT <200	91.5	132.0	249.5	107.5	150.0	257.5
NONPROFIT >200	171.0	202.5	464.0	200.0	339.0	480.0
UNIV/TEACH	294.0	399.0	1,024.0	300.0	500.0	969.0
FEDERAL/PUBLIC	98.0	134.0	286.5	98.0	134.0	362.0
PROPRIETARY	115.5	177.0	263.0	135.0	311.0	487.5
NONHOSPITAL	100.0	792.0	2,096.0	250.0	792.0	2,096.0
LAB AREA—PROCUREMENT/DISPATCH						
NONPROFIT <200	71.5	119.0	313.5	120.0	150.0	348.0
NONPROFIT >200	152.5	245.0	459.8	224.0	304.0	540.0
UNIV/TEACH	240.3	466.5	708.8	353.5	600.0	872.0
FEDERAL/PUBLIC	100.0	162.0	294.0	140.0	220.0	375.5
PROPRIETARY	90.0	193.0	300.0	90.0	232.0	350.0
NONHOSPITAL	149.0	323.0	1,035.0	200.0	286.5	1,085.3
LAB AREA—URINE AND FECES						
NONPROFIT <200	32.0	79.0	143.0	41.0	100.0	171.5
NONPROFIT >200	72.3	158.0	230.0	150.0	175.0	249.0
UNIV/TEACH	102.3	170.0	210.3	140.0	203.0	301.5
FEDERAL/PUBLIC	96.0	137.0	168.0	100.0	150.0	200.0
PROPRIETARY	58.5	100.0	131.0	58.5	100.0	237.5
NONHOSPITAL	65.0	100.0	2,817.0	65.0	150.0	3,400.0

● ANATOMIC PATHOLOGY WORK AREAS

	Actual 25th	Actual Median	Actual 75th	Required 25th	Required Median	Required 75th
LAB AREA—AUTOPSY/MORGUE						
NONPROFIT <200	243.0	347.5	409.0	282.5	394.5	437.0
NONPROFIT >200	333.5	518.5	727.3	349.0	544.0	715.5
UNIV/TEACH	529.5	838.0	1,232.5	532.5	870.0	1,293.0
FEDERAL/PUBLIC	420.0	540.0	840.0	443.3	544.5	772.5
PROPRIETARY	295.5	361.0	421.5	309.0	361.0	552.8
NONHOSPITAL	*****	*****	*****	*****	*****	*****
LAB AREA—ELECTRON MICROSCOPY						
NONPROFIT <200	162.0	258.0	395.3	177.0	350.0	420.0
NONPROFIT >200	384.5	800.0	1,166.0	435.0	800.0	1,357.5
UNIV/TEACH	350.0	558.0	1,303.0	618.8	715.0	1,217.0
FEDERAL/PUBLIC	*****	*****	*****	*****	*****	*****
PROPRIETARY	*****	*****	*****	*****	*****	*****
NONHOSPITAL	*****	*****	*****	*****	*****	*****
LAB AREA—HISTOLOGY/CYTOLOGY						
NONPROFIT <200	183.0	284.0	448.5	212.5	310.0	575.0
NONPROFIT >200	369.0	516.0	828.0	400.0	600.0	848.0
UNIV/TEACH	872.0	1,330.0	1,870.5	1,000.0	1,439.0	2,066.0
FEDERAL/PUBLIC	320.0	484.0	687.3	333.0	600.0	1,000.0
PROPRIETARY	304.0	457.5	755.8	317.5	498.5	808.0
NONHOSPITAL	646.0	1,088.0	2,315.0	646.0	1,088.0	2,600.0

* = No data or an insufficient amount of data

Table E.2

PERCENTAGE OF CLINICAL AND ANATOMIC SPACE OCCUPIED BY AREA

	Actual 25th	Actual Median	Actual 75th	Required 25th	Required Median	Required 75th
● CLINICAL PATHOLOGY WORK AREAS						
──────── LAB AREA—BLOOD BANK ────────						
NONPROFIT <200	5.7	9.0	12.8	6.7	9.6	12.8
NONPROFIT >200	8.0	10.5	16.0	7.9	11.3	15.1
UNIV/TEACH	8.0	10.3	12.4	8.0	11.4	13.2
FEDERAL/PUBLIC	6.5	9.7	13.4	6.1	8.3	13.0
PROPRIETARY	6.8	10.2	15.8	8.1	9.1	13.0
NONHOSPITAL	0.6	5.7	20.4	0.6	5.6	16.7
──────── LAB AREA—CHEMISTRY ────────						
NONPROFIT <200	28.1	34.0	48.1	28.1	34.8	45.2
NONPROFIT >200	26.5	34.6	41.2	25.2	32.8	38.4
UNIV/TEACH	22.2	31.7	39.5	22.9	28.7	35.4
FEDERAL/PUBLIC	26.0	35.9	40.9	30.3	34.7	42.4
PROPRIETARY	20.2	27.2	45.6	19.0	27.8	47.4
NONHOSPITAL	31.2	35.0	41.6	31.1	37.3	48.4
──────── LAB AREA—HEMATOLOGY/COAGULATION ────────						
NONPROFIT <200	9.2	13.8	18.9	10.5	14.2	17.2
NONPROFIT >200	11.9	13.9	16.7	11.1	13.5	17.5
UNIV/TEACH	9.6	13.2	16.8	10.3	13.8	17.2
FEDERAL/PUBLIC	10.3	13.6	18.9	11.6	14.8	19.7
PROPRIETARY	6.4	15.9	21.4	7.1	15.9	20.7
NONHOSPITAL	5.7	12.4	13.3	5.5	9.8	12.7
──────── LAB AREA—IMMUNOLOGY ────────						
NONPROFIT <200	2.0	3.6	7.3	2.9	4.7	6.5
NONPROFIT >200	2.7	4.5	6.4	2.6	4.2	6.3
UNIV/TEACH	3.2	5.6	9.4	3.5	6.3	10.0
FEDERAL/PUBLIC	2.8	5.6	7.0	2.4	3.1	6.6
PROPRIETARY	2.1	7.0	8.8	3.5	7.1	8.8
NONHOSPITAL	4.9	7.5	11.8	5.3	7.0	7.9
──────── LAB AREA—MICROBIOLOGY ────────						
NONPROFIT <200	9.0	13.3	20.9	9.1	15.2	21.1
NONPROFIT >200	13.7	18.3	23.1	15.9	19.1	22.9
UNIV/TEACH	13.3	19.0	21.8	15.0	19.5	24.8
FEDERAL/PUBLIC	15.8	22.3	30.3	15.6	20.1	27.1
PROPRIETARY	14.2	16.1	23.7	13.8	16.7	21.8
NONHOSPITAL	13.0	17.6	26.2	12.9	21.9	27.1

(continued)

Table E.2 (continued)	Actual 25th	Actual Median	Actual 75th	Required 25th	Required Median	Required 75th
LAB AREA—RADIOISOTOPES						
NONPROFIT <200	5.3	6.1	10.9	5.2	7.5	10.7
NONPROFIT >200	3.9	5.6	9.5	4.3	5.5	8.8
UNIV/TEACH	4.4	5.9	11.6	4.3	5.9	10.1
FEDERAL/PUBLIC	2.5	5.9	8.7	2.2	6.1	7.9
PROPRIETARY	2.7	5.4	10.1	2.5	6.5	11.5
NONHOSPITAL	4.7	12.6	23.1	6.8	12.5	19.5
LAB AREA—PROCUREMENT/DISPATCH						
NONPROFIT <200	4.4	7.5	13.9	5.9	7.9	15.9
NONPROFIT >200	4.1	6.7	10.0	5.0	7.1	10.0
UNIV/TEACH	4.0	6.0	8.7	4.8	6.3	10.3
FEDERAL/PUBLIC	4.1	7.0	9.1	4.1	6.0	8.2
PROPRIETARY	6.6	7.3	12.5	6.5	7.4	13.0
NONHOSPITAL	8.3	12.9	18.6	6.3	12.6	18.1
LAB AREA—URINE AND FECES						
NONPROFIT <200	2.2	4.8	6.9	2.6	4.5	6.7
NONPROFIT >200	2.0	3.5	5.0	2.4	3.6	4.9
UNIV/TEACH	1.4	2.4	3.4	1.4	2.8	4.2
FEDERAL/PUBLIC	3.3	3.8	7.1	1.7	3.4	6.7
PROPRIETARY	2.2	3.6	5.2	2.7	3.6	5.8
NONHOSPITAL	1.6	10.9	18.8	1.6	7.5	17.2

● ANATOMIC PATHOLOGY WORK AREAS

	Actual 25th	Actual Median	Actual 75th	Required 25th	Required Median	Required 75th
LAB AREA—AUTOPSY/MORGUE						
NONPROFIT <200	37.5	51.7	65.5	37.5	51.7	70.1
NONPROFIT >200	31.8	42.9	58.1	32.0	38.5	54.9
UNIV/TEACH	20.1	30.3	39.0	20.1	27.5	36.6
FEDERAL/PUBLIC	31.6	56.3	70.1	32.1	47.0	61.2
PROPRIETARY	28.1	39.4	70.0	28.7	39.2	64.5
NONHOSPITAL	11.4	29.7	48.0	11.4	29.7	48.1
LAB AREA—ELECTRON MICROSCOPY						
NONPROFIT <200	****	****	****	****	****	****
NONPROFIT >200	7.1	8.5	24.7	7.8	8.9	17.8
UNIV/TEACH	7.5	17.9	22.0	8.3	16.8	26.1
FEDERAL/PUBLIC	7.6	9.8	26.6	6.9	14.1	31.4
PROPRIETARY	****	****	****	****	****	****
NONHOSPITAL	****	****	****	****	****	****
LAB AREA—HISTOLOGY/CYTOLOGY						
NONPROFIT <200	37.8	55.3	78.0	38.9	51.1	68.6
NONPROFIT >200	35.6	51.9	64.1	35.6	54.2	63.6
UNIV/TEACH	35.4	49.2	62.3	34.8	46.8	62.5
FEDERAL/PUBLIC	23.1	37.6	46.6	24.6	35.5	54.8
PROPRIETARY	30.0	51.8	70.3	35.5	48.0	67.1
NONHOSPITAL	36.9	75.9	100.0	36.9	75.9	100.0

254

* = No data or an insufficient amount of data

Table E.3

AVAILABILITY AND NEED OF NONTEST PERFORMANCE AREAS IN 201
LABORATORIES EXPRESSED IN PERCENT

	Have Area	Would Like	Not Needed
ADMINISTRATION AREAS	87.06	0.50	12.44
Offices	94.03	0.50	5.47
Library	36.32	23.88	39.80
Conference Room(s)	43.78	24.38	31.84
Secretarial Space	90.55	1.99	7.46
Record Storage	74.13	10.45	15.42
Computer Room(s)	34.83	18.91	46.27
EDUCATIONAL AREAS	37.81	14.43	47.76
Classroom(s)	33.83	11.44	54.73
Demonstration Lab(s)	9.45	6.47	84.08
Photography	22.39	7.96	69.65
Research and Development	8.96	8.46	82.59
PATIENT SUPPORT AREAS	77.61	1.99	20.40
Waiting Room	76.12	11.94	11.94
Reception	60.70	7.46	31.84
Toilets	86.07	2.49	11.44
Examination Room(s)	34.83	9.45	55.72
EMPLOYEE SUPPORT AREAS	77.61	4.48	17.91
Lounge	61.19	20.40	18.41
Lockers	58.71	21.39	19.90
Toilets	83.08	6.97	9.95
Shower(s)	33.83	13.43	52.74
STORAGE AREAS	83.08	1.00	15.92
In Laboratory	87.56	5.47	6.97
Outside Laboratory	65.67	4.48	29.85
Janatorial	55.72	6.97	37.31
OTHER NONTEST AREAS	62.19	2.49	35.32
Refrigerators	74.63	2.49	22.89
Shipping	13.93	3.48	82.59
Animal Facilities	1.49	0.50	98.01

Table E.4

OPINIONS ON HOW CERTAIN FACTORS MAY AFFECT LABORATORY SPACE NEEDS EXPRESSED IN PERCENT

	Increase Area Needed	Decrease Area Needed	No Effect	Cannot Predict
HEALTH CARE PLANNING				
Nonprofit <200	48.3	6.9	41.4	3.4
Nonprofit >200	19.3	14.0	64.9	1.8
Univ/Teach	23.7	21.1	55.3	0.0
Federal/Public	38.2	11.8	47.1	2.9
Proprietary	28.6	21.4	42.9	7.1
Nonhospital Lab	28.6	14.3	57.1	0.0
CHANGE IN NUMBER OF TESTS				
Nonprofit <200	56.7	10.0	30.0	3.3
Nonprofit >200	36.8	19.3	38.6	5.3
Univ/Teach	50.0	19.4	22.2	8.3
Federal/Public	70.6	0.0	26.5	2.9
Proprietary	42.9	14.3	35.7	7.1
Nonhospital Lab	75.0	0.0	12.5	12.5
CHANGES IN METHODOLOGY				
Nonprofit <200	26.7	20.0	53.3	0.0
Nonprofit >200	27.1	25.4	44.1	3.4
Univ/Teach	22.9	25.7	42.9	8.6
Federal/Public	44.1	20.6	35.3	0.0
Proprietary	28.6	28.6	42.9	0.0
Nonhospital Lab	50.0	12.5	25.0	12.5
FUNCTIONS ADDED OR DROPPED				
Nonprofit <200	53.3	6.7	36.7	3.3
Nonprofit >200	40.4	12.3	36.8	10.5
Univ/Teach	45.7	11.4	28.6	14.3
Federal/Public	54.5	3.0	39.4	3.0
Proprietary	30.8	15.4	38.5	15.4
Nonhospital Lab	57.1	0.0	28.6	14.3
CHANGE IN NUMBER OF BEDS				
Nonprofit <200	60.0	3.3	33.3	3.3
Nonprofit >200	36.8	15.8	43.9	3.5
Univ/Teach	37.8	10.8	40.5	10.8
Federal/Public	54.5	0.0	45.5	0.0
Proprietary	57.1	14.3	28.6	0.0
Nonhospital Lab	****	****	****	****
CHANGE IN PATIENT MIX				
Nonprofit <L200	37.9	3.4	55.2	3.4
Nonprofit >200	40.4	3.5	52.6	3.5
Univ/Teach	43.2	5.4	45.9	5.4
Federal/Public	33.3	6.1	60.6	0.0
Proprietary	14.3	7.1	78.6	0.0
Nonhospital Lab	25.0	0.0	75.0	0.0

* = No data or an insufficient amount of data

Personnel (including satellite and special function laboratory personnel)

Each laboratory was asked to list their personnel by type and laboratory section. The results of this data are depicted in Figures E.11 through E.16. Abbreviations used are as follows:

BB — Blood Bank
CHM — Chemistry
HEM — Hematology and Coagulation
HIS — Histology and Cytology
IMM — Immunology
MIC — Microbiology
ISO — Radioisotopes (nuclear medicine)
PLB — Specimen procurement and dispatch
(phlebotomy)

URI — Urine and feces
ADM — Administrative
R&D — Research and development
CPTR — Computer/Data processing
OTH — Other
PhD — Doctoral-level personnel
TECH — Registered medical technologists
NR TECH — Nonregistered technologists
SEC — Secretaries and clerks

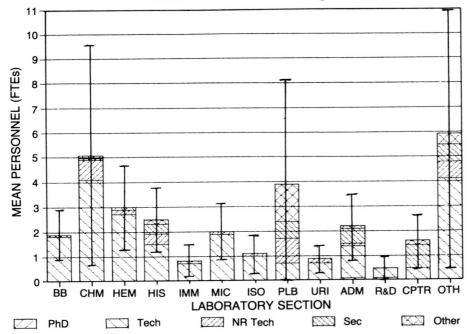

Fig. E.11   PERSONNEL BY LAB SECTION (NP <200)
Mean Values with 1 SD Range for Totals

257

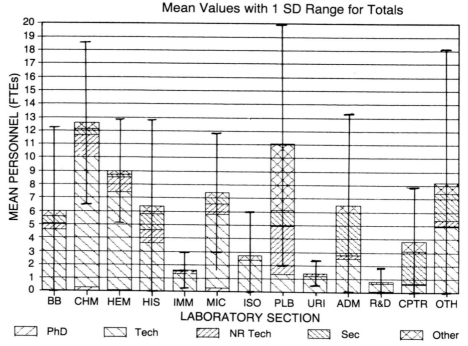

Fig. E.12   PERSONNEL BY LAB SECTION (NP >200)
Mean Values with 1 SD Range for Totals

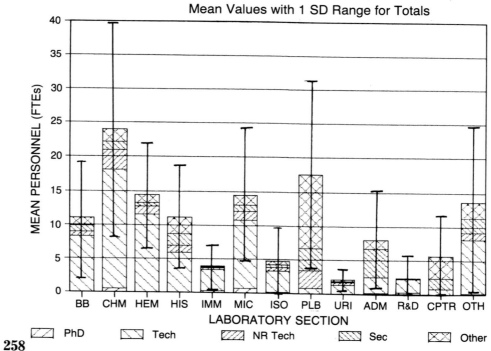

Fig. E.13   PERSONNEL BY LAB SECTION (UNIV/TEACH)
Mean Values with 1 SD Range for Totals

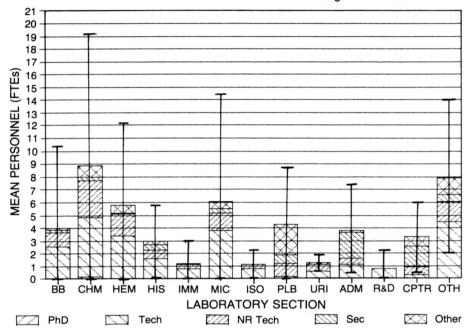

Fig. E.14 PERSONNEL BY LAB SECTION (FED/PUB)
Mean Values with 1 SD Range for Totals

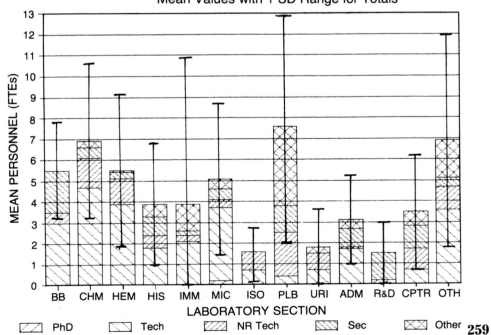

Fig. E.15 PERSONNEL BY LAB SECTION (PROPRIETARY)
Mean Values with 1 SD Range for Totals

259

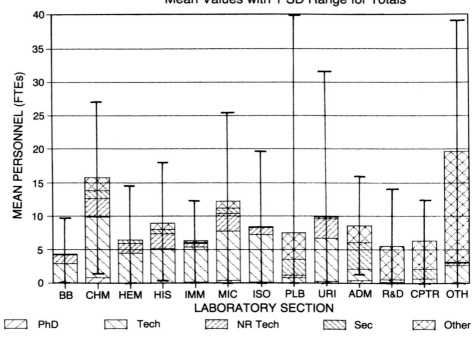

Fig. E.16 PERSONNEL BY LAB SECTION (NONHOSP)
Mean Values with 1 SD Range for Totals

Other personnel are also found in the laboratory. Their occurrence is shown in Figure E.17.

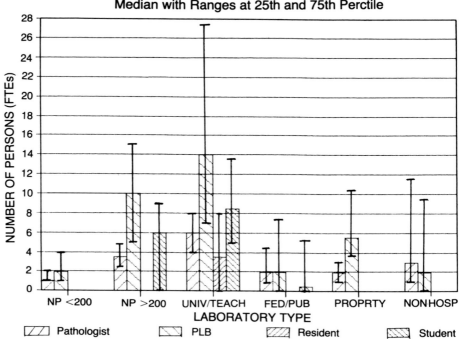

Fig. E.17 OTHER LAB PERSONNEL
Median with Ranges at 25th and 75th Perctile

Often when designing a laboratory it is useful to know the maximum number of personnel that may be working in the facility at any one time. This is helpful in determining requirements for restrooms, lounges, and other personnel support areas. The results by laboratory type are shown in Figure E.18.

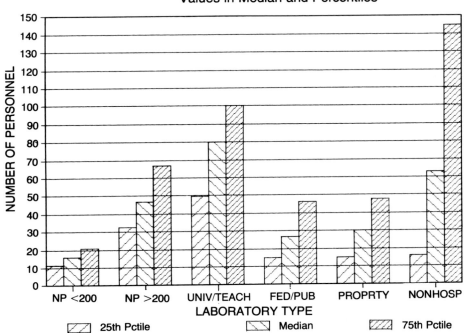

Fig. E.18 MAXIMUM PERSONNEL IN MAIN LAB AT ONE TIME
Values in Median and Percentiles

Laboratory Workload

The CAP Workload Recording Method is a management aid designed to measure effectively the productive time expended by technical, clerical, and aide staff performing procedures in the clinical laboratory. The generated data can assist in making decisions regarding space, staffing, equipment, and technical method selection.

The unit value per procedure, the core of the Method, is a measure of the technical, clerical, and aide time expressed in minutes required to complete a defined procedure once.

The total workload is the sum of all the products obtained by multiplying the total raw count for each individual procedure by its unit value. The total

261

raw count includes procedures performed on patient specimens, quality controls, and standard specimens as well as repeats.

The total unit value divided by the number of FTEs gives an approximation of personnel efficiency. For example, 45 units/hour/FTE would indicate that each FTE person is working 45 minutes each hour in actual test production. Because of the efficiency of some instrumentation and computerization, differences of efficiency may be seen between sections within a laboratory. A projection of required FTEs can be determined by dividing the total unit value by units/hour and dividing the answer by the number of hours per year each FTE works.

Some basic descriptive statistics by laboratory type are listed in Table E.5. The raw counts and unit values for participant laboratories are shown in Table E.6.

Table E.5

**ANNUAL LABORATORY WORKLOAD (RAW COUNT)
DESCRIPTIVE STATISTICS**

	25th Pctile	Median	75th Pctile
SPECIMENS COLLECTED			
NONPROFIT <200	19,664	49,275	63,560
NONPROFIT >200	60,000	89,615	132,275
UNIV/TEACH	89,129	153,069	231,499
FEDERAL/PUBLIC	35,519	52,000	128,097
PROPRIETARY	36,256	49,262	254,555
NONHOSPITAL	7,818	17,100	42,400
SPECIMENS SENT TO OUTSIDE LAB			
NONPROFIT <200	1,530	3,131	9,813
NONPROFIT >200	2,008	3,600	7,177
UNIV/TEACH	3,385	5,309	7,954
FEDERAL/PUBLIC	1,692	2,900	8,681
PROPRIETARY	1,900	3,719	5,081
NONHOSPITAL	280	2,872	15,250
INPATIENT PROCEDURES			
NONPROFIT <200	82,110	179,314	302,572
NONPROFIT >200	345,577	663,618	971,298
UNIV/TEACH	506,062	961,058	1,673,854
FEDERAL/PUBLIC	100,627	327,657	866,465
PROPRIETARY	138,427	225,291	48,6974
NONHOSPITAL	******	******	******

(continued)

262

Table E.7 (continued)	Raw Cnt 25th Pctile	Raw Cnt Median	Raw Cnt 75th Pctile	Unit Val 25th Pctile	Unit Val Median	Unit Val 75th Pctile
LAB AREA—RADIOISOTOPES						
NONPROFIT <200	95.0	100.0	100.0	94.5	100.0	100.0
NONPROFIT >200	76.5	95.0	100.0	95.0	96.5	100.0
UNIV/TEACH	72.3	100.0	100.0	76.8	100.0	100.0
FEDERAL/PUBLIC	0.0	96.0	100.0	0.0	94.0	99.0
PROPRIETARY	0.0	60.0	100.0	60.0	80.0	100.0
NONHOSPITAL	****	****	****	****	****	****
LAB AREA—PROCUREMENT/DISPATCH						
NONPROFIT <200	71.3	80.0	86.5	65.0	75.0	85.0
NONPROFIT >200	66.0	72.0	90.0	65.8	79.0	90.0
UNIV/TEACH	59.0	68.0	90.0	58.5	70.0	90.0
FEDERAL/PUBLIC	76.3	90.0	100.0	75.0	90.0	100.0
PROPRIETARY	52.0	60.0	75.0	54.5	60.0	77.5
NONHOSPITAL	****	****	****	****	****	****
LAB AREA—URINE AND FECES						
NONPROFIT <200	58.5	80.0	85.0	57.0	63.0	82.0
NONPROFIT >200	50.0	70.0	84.3	47.3	65.0	82.3
UNIV/TEACH	45.8	66.5	74.0	44.3	57.0	80.5
FEDERAL/PUBLIC	75.0	90.0	95.0	67.5	86.0	95.0
PROPRIETARY	39.0	60.0	62.0	39.0	49.5	60.0
NONHOSPITAL	****	****	****	****	****	****

* = No data or an insufficient amount of data

Regression Curves Relating Square Feet to Total Department Unit Value and FTEs

The following represents the most significant regression curves of a variety of cross correlations that were examined in the survey. The correlations and regressions that were examined included the following:

- correlations between raw counts and unit values per actual and required square feet, broken down by laboratory section and laboratory type—in most cases, unit values correlate better than raw counts, and required area is more closely related to workload than is actual area

- regressions with actual and required space as dependent variables, raw count and raw count squared as independent variables—scatter plots for these regressions, with two plots for each regression

- similar regressions using unit values instead of raw counts
- correlations between total patient days and actual and required square footage
- regressions of actual and required space versus total patient days and days squared including scatter plots as mentioned previously
- descriptive statistics for actual and required space per technologist by laboratory type (all sections combined) including correlations, regressions, and scatter plots as before
- actual and required square feet per technologist grouped by laboratory section (all laboratory types combined) including correlations, regressions, and scatter plots as before

As suspected, there is no single variable which will totally explain square footage needs in the laboratory. As one might expect, space does appear to be related to workload and the number of personnel who work in the area. In most of the studies done, space needs more closely correlated with required space as opposed to actual, and with unit values as opposed to raw count. This is because laboratorians more than anyone else are likely to know what space is required to perform a certain workload. Unit values, as opposed to raw count, are reflective of the methods and instrumentation used in test performance. Obviously, the methods and instruments used relate to space.

The best of all the cross correlations and regressions are presented in Table E.8 and Figures E.19 through E.22.

The Spearman formula for the correlation coefficient is the most appropriate for this type of data and p val is the test for the null hypotheses of the correlation. Nearly all correlations are in excess of 70 percent. Root MSE is the standard error of the regression and can be thought of as the standard deviation of values in square feet around the regression line. The strength of the regression is given by R-Square (the percentage of variability in the dependent variable that is explained by the independent variables, and by Root MSE). Prob>F is the test for the null hypothesis of the regression: no relationship between the dependent and independent variables.

It should be kept in mind that square footage is required square feet, e.g., that amount of space necessary to comfortably handle a particular workload, and in most cases is slightly greater than actual footage (Fig. E.10). The footage for a particular workload or FTE count should be considered a ballpark figure that represents only test performance area. It does not represent any nontest performance space.

Table E.8

TABLE OF VALIDITY VALUES FOR REGRESSION CURVES
(THE DEPENDENT VARIABLE IN ALL CASES IS SQ FT)

	Cor Coef	p Val	Rt MSE	R Square	Prob>F
───── FIGURE E.19—SQ FT VS UNIT VALUES ─────					
PHLEBOTOMY/DISPATCH	0.589	0.0001	315.1	0.2937	0.0001
HEMATOLOGY/COAGULATION	0.713	0.0001	559.1	0.5325	0.0001
HISTOLOGY/CYTOLOGY	0.705	0.0001	498.6	0.5449	0.0001
CHEMISTRY	0.735	0.0001	919.5	0.7102	0.0001
───── FIGURE E.20—SQ FT VS UNIT VALUES ─────					
BLOOD BANK	0.797	0.0001	348.7	0.8486	0.0001
IMMUNOLOGY	0.725	0.0001	252.5	0.5238	0.0001
MICROBIOLOGY	0.788	0.0001	600.8	0.6676	0.0001
───── FIGURE E.21—SQ FT VS FTEs ─────					
CHEMISTRY	0.713	0.0001	1153.9	0.5382	0.0001
HISTOLOGY/CYTOLOGY	0.733	0.0001	547.7	0.5435	0.0001
IMMUNOLOGY	0.801	0.0001	228.6	0.6496	0.0001
RADIOISOTOPES	0.789	0.0001	293.4	0.7607	0.0001
───── FIGURE E.22—SQ FT VS FTEs ─────					
BLOOD BANK	0.789	0.0001	403.7	0.7667	0.0001
HEMATOLOGY/COAGULATION	0.700	0.0001	620.0	0.3901	0.0001
MICROBIOLOGY	0.777	0.0001	915.1	0.5661	0.0001

Cor Coef = Spearman correlation coefficients

p Val = p value of correlation coefficient

Rt MSE = Standard error of the regression (Can be
thought of as the standard deviation of values
in square feet around the regression line.)

R Square = Variability of the area under the curve
(value × 100 = percent of variability of area
"explained" by the unit values or FTEs)

Prof>F = p value of regression curve

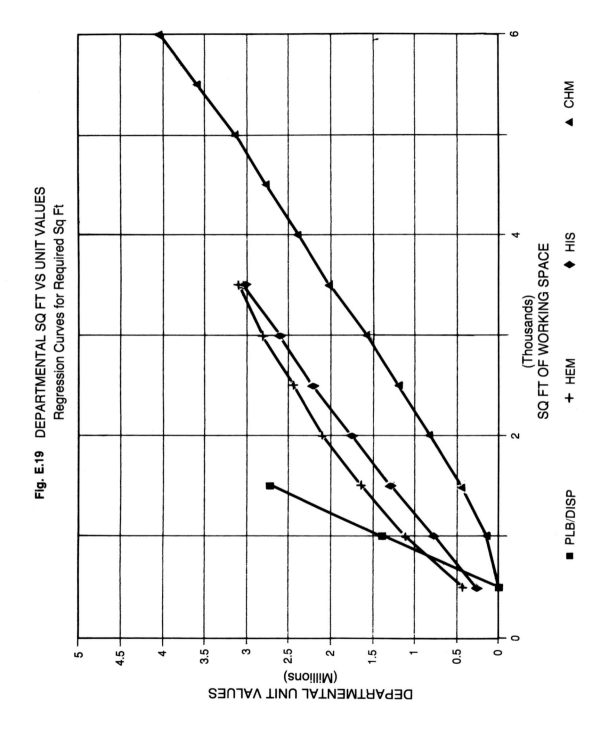

Fig. E.19   DEPARTMENTAL SQ FT VS UNIT VALUES
Regression Curves for Required Sq Ft

DEPARTMENTAL UNIT VALUES
(Millions)

SQ FT OF WORKING SPACE
(Thousands)

■ PLB/DISP   + HEM   ◆ HIS   ▲ CHM

Fig. E.20 DEPARTMENTAL SQ FT VS UNIT VALUES
Regression Curves for Required Sq Ft

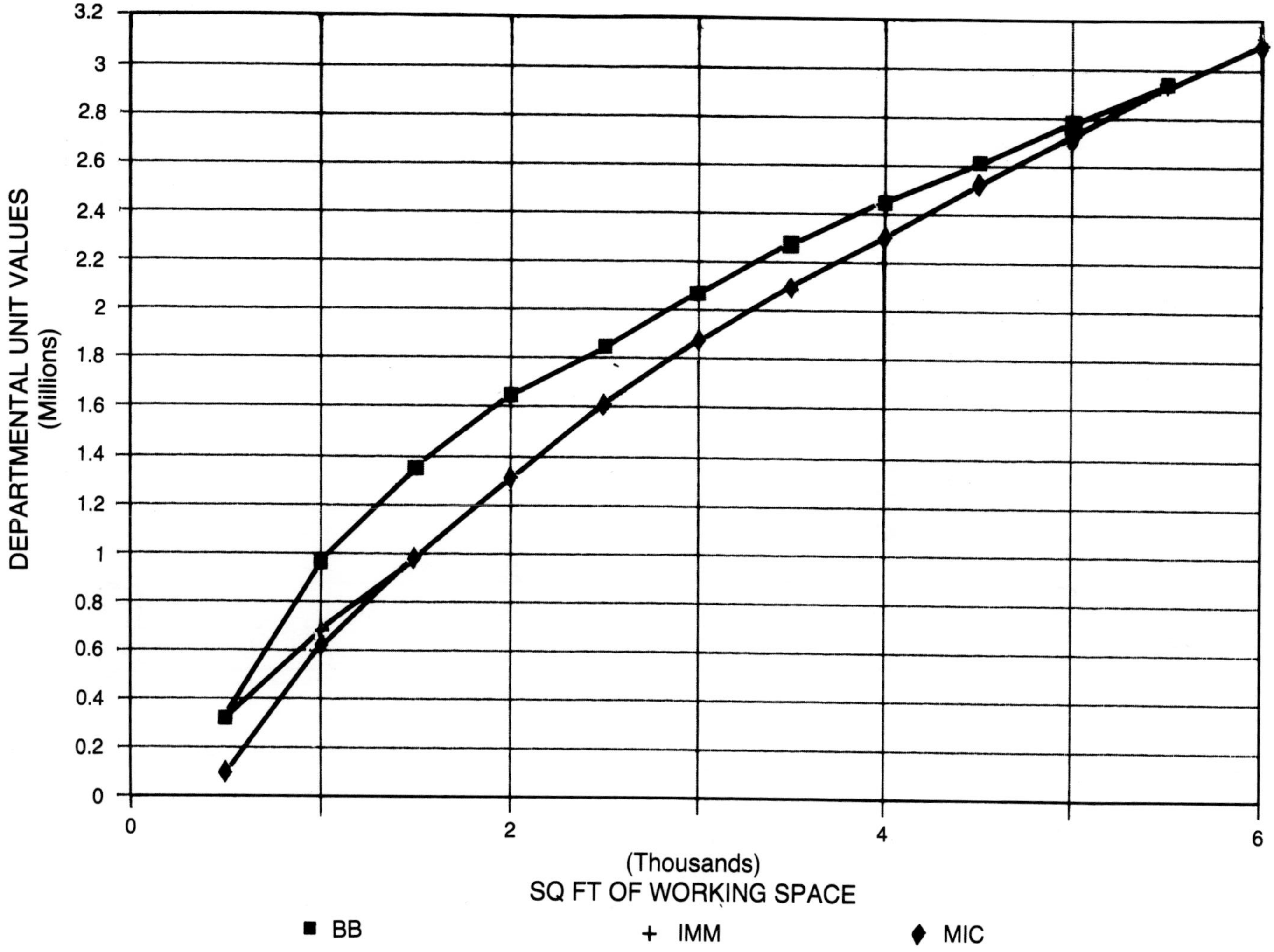

DEPARTMENTAL UNIT VALUES
(Millions)

SQ FT OF WORKING SPACE
(Thousands)

■ BB   + IMM   ◆ MIC

271

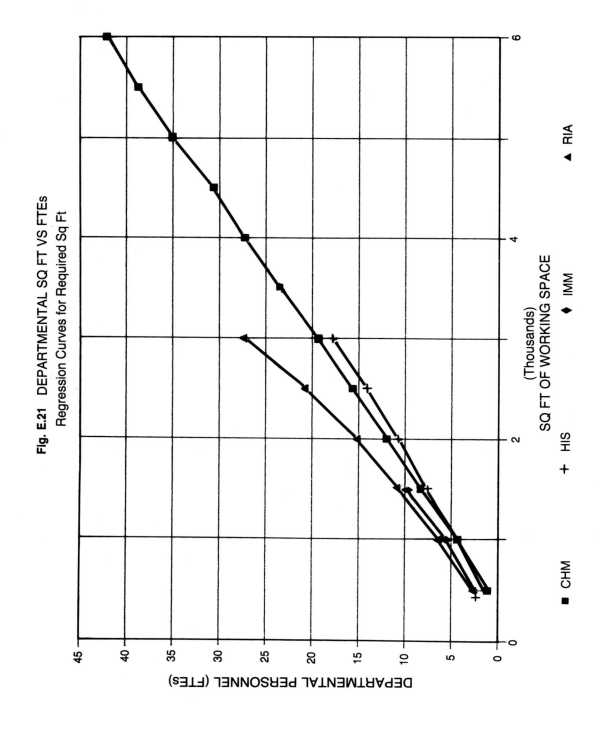

Fig. E.21 DEPARTMENTAL SQ FT VS FTEs
Regression Curves for Required Sq Ft

■ CHM   + HIS   ◆ IMM   ▲ RIA

SQ FT OF WORKING SPACE
(Thousands)

DEPARTMENTAL PERSONNEL (FTEs)

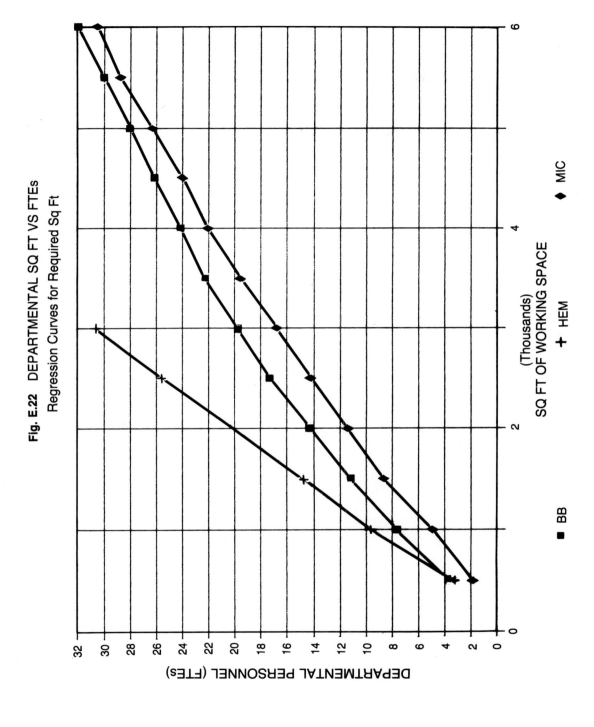

Fig. E.22 DEPARTMENTAL SQ FT VS FTEs
Regression Curves for Required Sq Ft

DEPARTMENTAL PERSONNEL (FTEs)

(Thousands)
SQ FT OF WORKING SPACE

■ BB   + HEM   ◆ MIC

273

INDEX

278